T0017282

MARIJUANA ON MY

Marijuana is on everyone's mind. Why do so many people enjoy it? What is it doing in our brains? Is it safe for everyone to use? What should we be telling our children? What are the benefits of medical marijuana? How does CBD live up to its hype? Does marijuana have spiritual power? And with so much conflicting information out there, how do we begin to make up our own minds about cannabis? *Marijuana on My Mind* is for anyone who has ever experienced the mystique of cannabis or wondered exactly how cannabis works. With over 40 years of clinical experience, Dr Timmen Cermak uses science to make sense of the endless debate between advocates and opponents of cannabis and provides answers to some of the greatest mysteries surrounding marijuana.

Dr Timmen Cermak is a retired addiction psychiatrist from California, with over 40 years' experience in clinical psychiatric practice. As Past-President of the California Society of Addiction Medicine, co-founder of the National Association for Children of Addiction and board member on California's Cannabis Advisory Committee, he brings extensive experience from the forefront of addiction medicine. He is an experienced author of books on the science of marijuana. His previous book, *From Bud to Brain: A Psychiatrists's View of Marijuana* (2020) was described by CHOICE Reviews as 'well written and researched' providing a 'wealth of science-based evidence'. Tim believes cannabis can be enjoyed safely by most people, with the correct guidance and precautions, and hopes *Marijuana on My Mind* will provide the public with the information they need to make educated and informed decisions about their own use.

"This is a fascinating account, or rather series of accounts, of cannabis – both medical and recreational – written from the perspective of a doctor with extensive clinical experience. The various effects of cannabis, both good and bad, are covered in a uniquely personal narrative that is both enjoyable and educational at the same time."

David Nutt FMedSci, author of *Cannabis (Seeing Through the Smoke): The New Science of Cannabis and Your Health.* Psychiatrist and Professor of Neuropsychopharmacology at Imperial College London.

"Beautifully written and cogently argued, *Marijuana on My Mind* interweaves the science and spirituality of cannabis in a book I that would recommend to patients, scientists, students, religious leaders, and anyone wanting to learn more about the science of cannabis, its impact on the human body, and its ramifications for the body politic. A fascinating read from a world expert."

Anna Lembke, MD, *New York Times* bestselling author of *Dopamine Nation: Finding Balance in the Age of Indulgence.*

"We needed a good, balanced, sensible and accessible book about cannabis and the brain, and here we have it. This book will help people understand the promise of cannabis as medicine, but also be aware of the potential dangers, particularly for the developing brain and for people with a predisposition to psychotic disorders such as schizophrenia. Readers will also appreciate that the hype about cannabis is not always backed up by the science, and that there is never a panacea for maladies of the mind."

David Castle, author of *Marijuana and Madness*, Professor of Psychiatry, University of Toronto

"In *Marijuana on My Mind*, the descriptor 'the science and mystique of cannabis' is aptly added to the title. To attempt to explain both the science of cannabinoids and touch upon the magic of this important plant would dissuade most from trying but Dr Cermak skillfully overcomes these challenges. This book is both enjoyable to read and also filled with information and interesting anecdotes that the lay public and the mental health clinician urgently need to understand. The first six chapters brilliantly lay the necessary scientific foundation to understand the cannabinoid systems. The next three chapters then tackle the important but frequently misunderstood topic of medical cannabis. Readers will especially appreciate Dr Cermak organizing the scientific evidence into strong and preliminary categories and spending time to visit the important topic of CBD. The final chapter introduces timely topics of interest and controversy for anyone interested in the science and public health implications of the uses of cannabis."

Steven James, Pharmaceutical Physician Executive

"Cermak has long been a student of cannabis and cannabinoids and has translated what he has learned into very readable texts. He is an excellent, clear writer – a wonderful teacher. He has also been a colleague of mine within professional societies, helping the California Society of Addiction Medicine and the American Society of Addiction Medicine develop evidence-based policy positions on cannabis. In *Marijuana on My Mind*, he uses his usual comfortable style of writing to share scientific detail as well as personal impressions from years of work as a psychiatrist, treating patients with addiction and others, and treating patients who have offered him their self-reports of their own use of cannabis and cannabinoids. His chapters on CBD are some of the most balanced and informative I have read. I have recommended Tim's previous books and I highly recommend this one."

Michael M. Miller, MD, DFASAM, DLFAPA, Past President, Amer Society of Addiction Medicine (ASAM)

"*Marijuana on My Mind* by Dr Timmen Cermak provides an honest, realistic, and personable account of cannabis. Dr Cermak skillfully and artfully combines history, society, science, and storytelling to explain how and why cannabis affects the mind, brain, and body. He provides a balanced perspective devoid of scare tactics, explaining the health effects of cannabis while also explaining the beneficial role that medical marijuana may have on some people struggling with various medical conditions. He also gives a wonderful explanation of addiction, and addresses the stigma of addiction. This book is perfect for adolescents, families, educators, healthcare clinicians, and anyone else interested in truly understand how and why cannabis affects the human body."

Bonnie Halpern-Felsher, PhD, Professor of Pediatrics/ Adolescent Medicine, Stanford University School of Medicine, and Founder and Executive Director, Cannabis Awareness and Prevention Toolkit

"*Marijuana on My Mind* provides an authoritative yet entertaining and readable guide to understanding cannabis, the most controversial plant of modern times. Beginning with a history of the discovery of the psychoactive effects of cannabis, Cermak dives deep into explicating how cannabis works on the brain, both how it produces the experience of being 'high' and sets the stage for the consequences of over-use, including addiction. The culture and mystique surrounding cannabis use are addressed, as are its established and potential medical uses, with a constant eye on separating fact from fiction. Particular attention is paid to the problem of the misuse or overuse of cannabis, including how to spot it, the underlying brain changes that lead to addiction, and the long-term consequences of use, as well as recovery from dependence on cannabis. The story of cannabis is told in a lively and engaging way, replete with numerous personal, clinical, and historical anecdotes, and illustrated with abundant pictures, figures, graphs, and charts. This book is now the most definitive one on cannabis available to the general population, and is highly recommended for anyone interested in an objective, scientific account of the effects of cannabis on human behavior."

Kim T. Mueser, PhD, Center for Psychiatric Rehabilitation, Professor of Occupational Therapy and Psychological and Brain Sciences, Boston University

Marijuana on My Mind

The Science and Mystique of Cannabis

TIMMEN L. CERMAK, MD

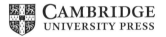

CAMBRIDGE
UNIVERSITY PRESS

University Printing House, Cambridge CB2 8BS, United Kingdom

One Liberty Plaza, 20th Floor, New York, NY 10006, USA

477 Williamstown Road, Port Melbourne, VIC 3207, Australia

314–321, 3rd Floor, Plot 3, Splendor Forum, Jasola District Centre,
New Delhi – 110025, India

103 Penang Road, #05–06/07, Visioncrest Commercial, Singapore 238467

Cambridge University Press is part of the University of Cambridge.

It furthers the University's mission by disseminating knowledge in the pursuit of
education, learning, and research at the highest international levels of excellence.

www.cambridge.org
Information on this title: www.cambridge.org/9781009010894
DOI: 10.1017/9781009024983

© Cambridge University Press 2022

First published 2022

Printed in the United Kingdom by TJ Books Limited, Padstow Cornwall

A catalogue record for this publication is available from the British Library.

ISBN 978-1-009-01089-4 Paperback

With deepest appreciation to my wife, Mary, who encourages, tolerates, and helps edit my writing habit.

CONTENTS

Science: The study of the physical and natural world through observation and experiment

Mystique: The aura of mystery, awe, and power surrounding someone or something

FOREWORD

I first met Tim in the early 1990s through our mutual professional involvement with the California Society of Addiction Medicine (CSAM) where we have both served as past presidents. I helped found the CSAM organization at a time when addiction was a crime and physicians were subject to arrest for treating addicts at the community level.

Not only a well-regarded practicing psychiatrist, Tim had also become CSAM's cannabis expert, following the basic science and clinical literature and sharing his insights with the medical community through his many lectures on cannabis. I was aware of his reputation as a compassionate caregiver and knowledgeable addiction psychiatrist, as we personally connected when he came to the aid of a family member of mine who needed help navigating the rocky road to recovery.

As a still-practicing addiction medicine physician, my own interest in Cannabis Culture, drug use, and its effects on individuals and society at large has always been a part of my medical career, and led me to open the Haight Ashbury Free Clinic during the Summer of Love in 1967. Our mission at the clinic was to treat the flocks of people who poured into San Francisco and desperately needed access to affordable and non-judgmental healthcare. We quickly became ground zero for treating a myriad of drug use issues, including addiction, and even established a safe space in the clinic called the "Calm Center," to help people come down from bad acid trips.

During the Summer of Love, the Haight was flooded with many drugs: speed, hallucinogens such as LSD and psilocybin mushrooms, and, of course, marijuana (also referred to as cannabis today). Marijuana quickly became a symbol of this hippie revolution as many embraced a new philosophy of "better living through chemistry." We saw many chronic pot users in the clinic who suffered from anxiety, paranoia, and impaired motivation, but these symptoms were masked by other more powerful drugs being used. In this way, the presence of marijuana was downplayed and its long-term effects were not really understood at the time.

People openly smoked pot everywhere, but it was risky. If caught smoking or holding, you could be fined and/or face up to 10 years in jail, as possession and marijuana use were illegal and considered a felony offense. Back then, the police were very hostile to the throngs of drug users (which included anti-war protesters) and conducted many raids, once arresting over 200 hippies at one time.

Marijuana's place in society has undergone a seismic shift since the 1960s, as this taboo, counterculture drug has now spread into the mainstream through legalization and medical use, not only in California but across the USA. However, its cultural acceptance for recreational and social use, similar to smoking a cigarette or drinking a beer in public, brings a host of issues, especially as today's cannabis strains are so much more potent than what was smoked in the past. In the medical field, we are now seeing cannabis addiction issues and rampant use among teens, with potentially deleterious, long-term consequences on the developing adolescent brain.

There is still so much to understand about the effects of cannabis on the mind and body, as well as its potential medical uses, and there is no better person to bridge the gap between scientific knowledge and public understanding than the author of the pivotal book you are holding in your hands. *Marijuana on My Mind: The Science and Mystique of*

Cannabis has been written for the general public, synthesizing decades of research, personal observations, clinical cases, and current trends into an accessible and profound resource on the facts and continued allure of cannabis.

Tim is no stranger to writing about cannabis. In addition to his studies and lectures, his previous book on the subject, *From Bud to Brain: A Psychiatrist's View of Marijuana*, summarized the science of cannabis for health professionals. And now with *Marijuana on My Mind*, everyone can benefit from his dedicated, balanced perspective and expert insights. From the very first chapter ("The Science and Mystique of Cannabis"), this book guides readers through the complex issues surrounding Cannabis Culture, including its history, links to spirituality, medical use, addiction, and public health and political concerns. By highlighting a thematic case example for each chapter, Tim makes the science personal and understandable, breaking down the issues vividly. Of particular value is the information he shares on the new advances in understanding cannabis chemistry, as well as the future of cannabis.

My two favorite chapters were Chapter 11 ("When Addiction Hijacks the Brain's Reward System") and Chapter 12 ("Adolescents and Cannabis") as they reflect and illuminate both my own research and my efforts as a physician treating teens addicted to cannabis. I believe that all readers will connect to this groundbreaking work as *Marijuana on My Mind* speaks to everyone – whether you are a light to moderate cannabis user, heavy smoker, curious layperson, concerned parent, addiction specialist, or medical professional. I will definitely be recommending this book to my patients and their families.

Tim combines science and his medical background with a description of his personal experience with marijuana as a young man to make him the perfect conduit to put the cannabis world in perspective. Knowing Tim well and admiring his many accomplishments, I recommend all who are interested in the complexities of cannabis chemistry and culture to read his informative and entertaining book.

David E. Smith, MD, DFASAM, FAACT
Founder, Haight Ashbury Free Medical Clinics
Past President, California Society of Addiction Medicine (CSAM)
Past President and Diplomate, American Society of Addiction Medicine (ASAM)
Current Chair of Addiction Medicine and Medical Quality Assurance Committee, Muir Woods
Medical Director, Avery Lane Treatment Center for Women
Co-author of *Unchain Your Brain: 10 Steps to Breaking the Addictions that Steal Your Life*.

1 THE SCIENCE AND MYSTIQUE OF CANNABIS

John agreed to an evaluation of his cannabis use to appease his mother. The 10th grader cautiously acknowledged experimenting with cannabis after his best friend had been given some pot by his older brother. John asked his friend for a joint and they had smoked together half a dozen times over the past 4 months. He sheepishly admitted liking marijuana, but he also knew pot carried some vague risk for people his age. His mother was terrified when she saw her son looking at websites about cannabis, but when confronted, he was honest with his parents about his use. After talking with John, I wasn't concerned that he was in any real danger. I taught him the signs of using cannabis too frequently, and we reviewed the reasons why he should delay use until he was a few years older.

John's parents had completely opposite experiences with cannabis, so it was no surprise that they held differing opinions on John's use. His mother, Carol, had watched helplessly as her older brother began smoking cannabis all day, every day, eventually dropping out of college and developing a serious addiction to harder drugs. Naturally, she was panicked by John's interest in marijuana. His father, William, had smoked marijuana on most weekends during his college years and felt it opened his mind in helpful ways, but he had lost interest in it soon after graduation. He dismissed his son's cannabis use as just a passing phase. I tried to soothe Carol's fears while helping William understand the difference between the weaker marijuana he used and the much *stronger cannabis available today, as well as how John's younger age put him at increased risk. They both wanted to know the best way to respond to John's use. I encouraged them to keep the conversation going so John didn't have to hide his interest, to trust their son's current judgment, and to learn as much as they could about the science of cannabis.*

"What can we read to educate ourselves?" they asked.

I didn't know what to tell them. Everything published at the time was based more on opinion than scientific fact and either strongly promoted or demonized cannabis.

So, I wrote the following book to help people like John, Carol, and William.

I have been curious about cannabis from the first moment it altered the texture of my experience in 1967, when I was only 22 years old. I was fascinated by how a simple plant, a "weed" that grows in the wild nearly everywhere, could change my experience of the world so dramatically. What did its chemistry do to my brain to make me feel so comfortable, relaxed, hungry, and spellbound by even the smallest details? How did it slow time and make the world look so fresh and new? And how did it vivify flavors and music, sending their sensations throughout my whole body? Even the seeds-and-stems, 3 percent THC marijuana of the 1960s could do all this without the numbing fogginess or blistering hangover I experienced with alcohol. I wanted to understand what was happening that made me feel so different, and what it all meant.

There were no believable answers to these questions available in 1967. Some of my friends gravitated toward mystical explanations during what they called the Age of Aquarius. They believed that cannabis possessed numinous qualities, suggesting a divine spirit dwelt within its buds. Consuming the plant supposedly transferred this spiritual energy into humans. Such ancient beliefs were widely held when the world seemed infused with spirits. Christian ritual continues to speak of the transfiguration of bread and wine into a spiritual force that can infuse the faithful who ingest it. Despite the sense of awe I felt following a good joint, the notion that ingesting cannabis transfers spiritual energy struck me as more metaphorical than factual. During my senior year of college, I switched from studying philosophy to pursue a career in psychiatry. As a result, I wanted to know more about what rigorous scientific research tells us about cannabis and the brain.

One solid fact about cannabis had been firmly established by that time. The identity and structure of cannabis's main psychoactive chemical – THC – had been discovered 3 years earlier, in 1964. We all mastered THC's complicated full name, Δ^9-tetrahydrocannabinol, and we repeated it endlessly, as though chanting this scientific term would give us understanding. The truth was that we still knew nothing about what THC does once it enters the brain. What *does* THC do in the brain to change our experience in its unique and characteristic ways? Can it be used safely? If so, how? I was eager to know more, but the understanding I sought was still almost three decades away.

While scientists were slowly grinding away in their laboratories to unlock the mysteries of cannabis, its recreational use rapidly gained popularity in America, despite increasingly harsh prison sentences during the politically motivated War on Drugs. Law enforcement drew no distinction between classifications of drugs. "Illicit" drugs were all lumped together and outlawed. Illegal is illegal, and the criminal justice system was the hammer that treated everyone using an illegal drug as a nail. Because cannabis was the most frequently used illicit drug, more users of cannabis were arrested and imprisoned than heroin or cocaine users. One drug enforcement agent wryly explained his enthusiasm for busting pot smokers by noting that they do not shoot back as often as users of harder drugs. Racial disparities pervaded the enforcement of cannabis prohibition during the War on Drugs, leading to disproportionate rates of arrest and imprisonment of minorities. Still, more and more people tried cannabis, and many continued using it. Today, more than half of Americans have used cannabis at least once. General acceptance of cannabis in American culture has led to the phrase "social use" gradually replacing "recreational use" to parallel language describing casual alcohol consumption.

The cultural acceptance of cannabis received a significant boost when California relegalized its medical use in 1996 after 59 years of prohibition. This policy reversal resulted from an unlikely coalition of advocates for the compassionate use of marijuana, including caregivers of AIDS patients, drug policy reformers opposed to the drug war's harsh treatment of drug users, aging hippies, grandmothers on chemotherapy, political radicals, scofflaws, future entrepreneurs, and marijuana advocates who saw its medical use as poking the camel's nose under the tent toward full legalization. Tactically, medical marijuana was the greatest Trojan horse since Troy. To the surprise of many, the National Academies of Sciences, Engineering, and Medicine issued a report in 2017 documenting the proven benefits of medical cannabis. Today, the future looks brighter than ever for developing safe and effective cannabis-based medicines for a variety of diseases.

I abandoned my quest for answers to the mysteries of how marijuana works while America was passing through decades of its punitive approach to cannabis. I had also decided that meaningful answers did not lie in repeating its use. After finishing medical school, I served as a general practitioner in the Indian Health Service, and then began psychiatry training at Stanford University. Although I tried my hand at research in a neurophysiology laboratory for a couple of years, I soon discovered that my personality is more suited to clinical work. I like talking to people more than performing repetitive experiments with laboratory animals. I was particularly drawn to addiction medicine. Strange as it may seem, I found working with alcoholics to be comfortable and fascinating, largely because my own father had suffered from alcoholism. For the next 20 years, I focused on the lasting impact a parent's alcoholism has on their child's personality. It was a personal exploration, but at the same time, I helped bring attention to a forgotten and neglected population by cofounding the National Association for Children of Alcoholics in 1982 (now the National Association for Children of Addiction). NACoA continues to raise awareness and advocate for services for those affected by familial addiction.

An Avalanche of Scientific Discoveries

Lightning struck when I least expected it. I heard the late Billy Martin (a professor at Virginia Commonwealth University, not the baseball manager) speak at a meeting of the California Society of Addiction Medicine (CSAM) in 1996. His lecture summarized the scientific discoveries about cannabis and the brain that had recently emerged from research laboratories around the globe, and I learned that researchers had begun solving the mysteries as early as 1988 that had intrigued me since the late 1960s. Monumental discoveries with far-reaching implications had proven that our brains are wired to respond to cannabis. THC, which is found exclusively in cannabis, produces its effect by mimicking our brain's natural chemistry and enhancing certain brain functions. This is analogous to putting high-octane fuel in your car or adding power assist to the brakes, additions that energize the normal function of the engine and brakes, respectively. Being high is the result of THC's mimicry of natural chemistry and its subsequent impact on the brain's chemical systems. To better understand cannabis, I first needed to learn more about the brain and how it typically functions. What parts of the brain are thrown into overdrive and out of normal equilibrium by THC? How do these changes lead to the experience of being high?

I was afire with excitement when I realized there was far more to know about cannabis than I had realized. Although I had been reading clinical research about cannabis use, I had not been following the basic laboratory science literature. Clinical literature describes research on patients – people who are negatively impacted by their cannabis use. Basic science research delves more deeply into the minute details of molecules and nerve cells, and the findings are published in dense journal articles that are difficult to decipher and almost impossible to find outside medical libraries. At the time of the CSAM conference, there was still no recognition or understanding of cannabis dependence in the clinical literature. Scientific literature, however, had already reported changes in the brain that were characteristic of addiction, caused by frequent cannabis use. I left Martin's lecture committed to learning as much as I could from journals not usually read by practicing doctors.

Fate conspired to open a path for me to study the basic science of cannabis. A couple of weeks after the conference, the California public was scheduled to vote on the Compassionate Use Act to legalize medical cannabis. At the society's business meeting, I naively asked if CSAM had taken any position on the proposition, only to discover that our public policy committee had not even discussed the issue. I soon found out that whoever asks a question will be recruited to find the answer, and I became the unofficial cannabis guy for CSAM. My first task was to write background papers on what the scientific literature said about the potential medical benefits of cannabis and the special risks of cannabis use by adolescents. For the next two and a half decades, I conducted a monthly survey of both clinical and basic science literature in pursuit of answers.

I have learned so much, but I also understand that science never gives us ultimate answers. Those are left for theologians and philosophers. Science is much better at continuing to push the frontiers of knowledge until the next layer of questions is revealed. For example, when scientists discovered that THC mimics the brain's natural chemistry, they next needed to examine the normal function of the THC-like chemicals discovered in our brain.

How do these THC-like chemicals typically function? Where are they concentrated? Why does our brain chemistry resemble cannabis? Or should we ask why the chemistry of cannabis resembles our brain? The first two questions have been answered, while the last two still remain dangling.

Science: The Public Realm

I first studied the public and private realms of the human experience in a freshman humanities class. Science exists in the public realm, where facts are objective realities, while our direct, subjective experience lies in the private realm. We all live in both realms simultaneously. For example, when asked about the drive from San Francisco to Los Angeles, one person may say it is a ghastly long way, while another may say they breeze between the two cities easily. Subjective experience exists in the private recesses of our mind. We can communicate about the private realm, but no one can prove whether the drive feels long or short, and disagreements cannot be resolved. However, everyone agrees that the two cities are 381 miles (~613 km) apart because objective, concrete facts exist in the public realm. Whether you experience the drive as long or short, your car will need enough gas to drive 381 miles.

My previous book, *From Bud to Brain: A Psychiatrist's View of Marijuana*, detailed the science of cannabis and focused on the public realm. I wanted to provide health professionals and educators with the objective facts about cannabis, complete with a god-awful number of footnote references. I felt the book was necessary to give doctors, nurses, therapists, and educators relevant answers to patients' questions about the safety of social/recreational cannabis use and its potential medical benefits. As soon as I finished that book, I knew I had to turn my attention toward the general public, to answer Carol and William's question about where they could find clear and understandable information about cannabis. The public's scientific literacy about cannabis remains confused by biased and misleading websites and is limited by the lack of a dependably accurate source of understandable scientific information.

Responsible personal and policy decisions require a solid foundation of science literacy about cannabis and the brain. The importance of possessing greater science literacy is only increasing as more people across the USA and around the world gain legal access to cannabis. In the words of astrophysicist and popular science commentator Neil deGrasse Tyson, "Science literacy is an outlook that you bring with you in your daily walk through life. It's a lens through which you look that affects how you see the world." Science literacy means knowing more than just the basics; it means understanding the key scientific concepts and methods that create confidence in the facts established by scientists. It helps us make healthy personal decisions and participate in reasoned political debate in an increasingly complex world.

Science is a communal process. Scientific facts require corroboration from others using the same methods for observing the world. While science may be advanced by an individual's private experience, such as how August Kekulé's dream of a snake devouring its own tail gave him an intuitive understanding of the cyclic structure of benzene, intuition becomes scientific fact only after others are able to reproduce the result. The path of science relies on the transparency of methods for making objective measurements, followed by confirmation by others. The goal is to minimize opinion and unconscious bias by subjecting observations to the scrutiny of others' skepticism.

Accurate measurement is at the core of the scientific method. Nineteenth-century physicist Lord Kelvin said, "When you can measure what you are speaking about, and express it in numbers, you know something about it. When you cannot express it in numbers, your knowledge is of a meager and unsatisfactory kind. It may be the beginning of knowledge, but you have scarcely in your thoughts advanced to the stage of science." Once something is measured, scientific research and experimentation can begin in earnest.

Experience: The Private Realm

Understanding how cannabis influences brain chemistry is fascinating, but science is only one part of the cannabis story. It is a mistake to believe science is the only lens for observing the world. While a book intended for the general public needs to translate complex scientific concepts about cannabis and the brain into simple terms, it also needs to explore the mystique this plant holds for many people. The private realm contains the meaning people ascribe to their experience of being high and motivates the Cannabis Culture that has developed around cannabis use. This culture often ignores or cherry-picks scientific facts about cannabis because understanding the basic mechanics of the plant's effect on the brain is of little relevance to the metaphysical meaning many see in the cannabis experience. Ultimately, both the science and mystique of cannabis must be explored to fully understand the role it plays in today's world.

While our individual experience of meaning, beauty, morality, and spirituality is entirely subjective, it often holds more sway than scientific fact. Direct experience of our existence as part of the infinite universe is highly individual and ineffable, but it is as important to our sense of identity as an intellectual understanding of our evolution from earlier primates. Scientific fact and subjective experience are different lenses, each perhaps more associated with the left and right sides of the brain, respectively. Each perspective is valuable, just as both feet are necessary to walk forward into the world. Using only one foot while ignoring the other leads to walking in circles, a sensation of motion that leads nowhere. Science alone lacks humanistic meaning and values, while subjective experience alone can be unmoored from the concrete world we all share. Ignoring the concrete facts established by science increases the risk of experiencing negative consequences from cannabis use. However, our private realm never resonates as strongly with scientific facts as it does with a good story or emotional anecdote about cannabis.

Overview of *Marijuana on My Mind*

A book is different from the Internet, which tends to present information in factoids. This is useful when looking for quick answers to specific questions, but it often leads to being able to recite facts without understanding how we know they are true. This thin layer of knowledge is useful for Trivial Pursuit, like knowing the scientific name for THC without having the slightest understanding of how THC works, but factoids lack the depth needed to achieve meaningful understanding. Books can reveal the bigger picture and establish a basis for the facts used to support its conclusions.

Marijuana on My Mind tells the story of the impact of cannabis on both the brain and the mind. It is best to read the book sequentially rather than skip between chapters, as each chapter is built upon information already presented. The next three chapters describe the basic mechanism of cannabis interactions with the brain. Chapter 2 provides the background needed to understand the cannabis plant and the mind-altering products extracted and manufactured from it. Chapter 3 describes the basic architecture and function of brain cells, called neurons, in order to make sense of how THC alters communication between cells. Chapter 4 puts all this information together to trace how THC's impact on the brain results in the experience of being high.

The next two chapters put the impact of cannabis on society into perspective. Chapter 5 explores how many people use cannabis and how often they use it. To better understand the epidemiology of cannabis use, the chapter compares patterns of use and attitudes about alcohol and cannabis. Chapter 6 examines the lens of Cannabis Culture and its appreciation for the mystique of cannabis. Grasping the full meaning of the mental effects of cannabis requires exploring why mystics have used cannabis in their spiritual practices for millennia. The chapter takes a serious look at the important role the plant plays in the spiritual life of Cannabis Culture.

Cannabis Culture deserves much of the credit for keeping awareness of the medical benefits of cannabis alive and reawakening California's interest in legalizing its use. The next three chapters are devoted to exploring the evidence supporting the use of medical cannabis. Chapter 7 reviews the history of medical cannabis, places the value of anecdotal evidence into proper perspective, and assesses the medical benefits for which substantial scientific proof exists. Chapter 8 explores a wider range of benefits for which there is considerable suggestive evidence that does not yet rise to the level of proof needed for acceptance by the general medical community. Understanding the impact of cannabis on the brain and body lends credibility to many scientists' belief that cannabis-based medications will gain acceptance as treatment for a wide array of diseases. Finally, Chapter 9 explores the unique qualities of CBD in order to separate fact from fad and explore its legitimate medical use.

All medications have potential side effects, and this is true for cannabis as well, whether it is used to treat illness or for social/recreational pleasure. The next couple of chapters explain two overlapping negative effects of continuing to use cannabis beyond the brain's ability to maintain its normal chemical balance. Chapter 10 focuses on the five signs that indicate cannabis is being used too frequently. Awareness of these signs is essential for using cannabis safely. Chapter 11 explains the changes in the brain that lead to cannabis addiction. Although many in the Cannabis Culture strongly resist the idea that cannabis can be addictive, scientific evidence proves that it is. Accepting this inconvenient truth goes a long way toward knowing how to use cannabis without becoming addicted.

Not everyone recognizes the signs of using cannabis too frequently or avoids addiction. This is especially true for adolescents. Most people understand that cannabis can harm the developing brain, but few understand the significance of this catchy phrase. Chapter 12 lays out the reasons adolescents become addicted to drugs, including cannabis, more often and more quickly than adults. Chapter 13 explores the subtle but pervasive effects of long-term, daily (or near daily) cannabis use. A large body of evidence reveals a wide range of measurable intellectual and emotional impacts on adults who use cannabis frequently, whether overt addiction exists or not. Chapter 14 explores the process of quitting cannabis once an individual decides it has become a problem. It answers the following questions: What can be expected of recovery? When is treatment useful? What does treatment look like? How can family members help a loved one, especially a child, who is harmfully involved with cannabis?

During the COVID-19 pandemic, we all gained a new appreciation for the importance of a robust public health policy. Chapter 15 looks at the impact of public policies governing cannabis on both society and individuals. As medical cannabis becomes widely available in the USA and full legalization expands, it is increasingly important for the public to understand the complexity and difficulty the states face in regulating the cannabis industry. In Chapter 15, I describe my experience on the California Cannabis Advisory Committee to shed light on some of the issues legalization must confront.

Finally, what will be the future of cannabis? The Epilogue speculates on future developments for cannabis, medically, recreationally, and as the leading edge of a more humane approach to all drug use. Well-balanced natural cannabinoid brain chemistry is essential for optimal health, so exploring non-cannabis ways to enhance our natural THC-like brain chemistry will become a part of general wellness programs. As access increases, knowledge of how to use cannabis safely will be widespread, although still not always attended to. Whatever changes occur in the future of cannabis, human nature is likely to remain the same. The impulse to overuse a good thing will continue to produce harm.

Three addenda offer additional assistance to readers: a glossary, suggestions for further reading, and the source references for the included illustrations. For ease of reading, I have not included footnotes throughout the text. The Further Reading section provides additional resources to expand and document selected topics of interest. More extensive and detailed references can be found in *From Bud to Brain: A Psychiatrist's View of Marijuana*.

Conclusion

My first experience with cannabis left me with an enormous number of questions with no clear answers. The following chapters use plain language and simple scientific concepts to walk readers through the most interesting and substantiated answers available today. In order to provide the most reliable information possible, my greatest goal is objectivity. The bottom line is that cannabis *can* be used safely by most adults, but only if they do not get so lost in the pleasure and awe that they fail to respect their brain's finite ability to maintain a healthy chemical balance. Understanding what is currently known about cannabis and the brain will help readers make healthy and informed decisions. I hope this information satisfies and stimulates your curiosity as much as it has mine.

While there are a few black and white truths in life, we mostly inhabit the vast area in between these two extremes of certainty. Welcome to the beauty, freedom, and responsibility of the gray zones explored in this book.

2 THE PLANT, ITS HISTORY, AND ITS PRODUCTS

Martin was an intelligent and cocky young man whose father hoped therapy would help him cut down his cannabis use and mature enough to take over the family's successful road construction business. Martin only wanted me to help him get away from his father. He was convinced that his cannabis use was part of a healthy life, and he constantly tried to prove that he knew more about the plant than I did. In fact, he did know far more than I about the latest varieties of cannabis and new methods of cultivation. I allowed him to be the expert about what was available at his favorite dispensaries, while I was more interested in hearing how it altered his mind. He dismissed my concerns as those of an old man, but he tolerated me because he liked to argue. In the end, he didn't change his cannabis use, but he did gradually develop a better relationship with his family and returned home to manage the business when his father suffered a heart attack.

I saw an interesting and warm man beneath Martin's arrogant exterior, and he knew I liked him. He arrived at our final session with a small, neatly wrapped gift and insisted I open it immediately. Inside the box was a dried cannabis bud resting on a royal purple, velvet pillow. It looked like a giant, withered, alien Brussels sprout (Figure 2.1). Martin proudly pronounced, "This is the best bud I have ever found, with a really spiritual high. You should know about it."

I told Martin I appreciated the thought and knew he was giving me something precious, then closed the box and placed it back on

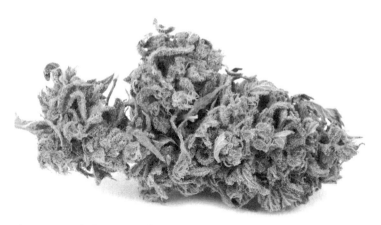

Figure 2.1 Dried cannabis flower, also called marijuana or bud.

the end table next to his chair. I handed it back to him as we shook hands when he left my office, but then I found it on the floor just outside my door when the next patient arrived. As I picked up the box, I said, "Drug reps are always leaving me little trinkets," but I knew Martin's gift was more heartfelt than the usual swag left by drug companies. I eventually encased the bud in a plexiglass cube and set it on my bookshelf beside the Freud action figure another patient had given me.

The History Behind Today's Cannabis

The dried bud Martin ceremoniously presented to me descended from a unique plant with a history that long predates humanity. Cannabis first emerged nearly 30 million years ago on the high-altitude, arid grasslands of Tibet, where it diverged from hops, its closest relative best known for flavoring beer. Cannabis became unique among Earth's vegetation by developing chemical compounds never seen before. Like all flowering plants, different varieties of cannabis evolved, some with revolutionary new chemistry and some without. *Marijuana on My Mind* focuses on those varieties that developed medicinal and mind-altering properties. The varieties of cannabis lacking this chemistry, called hemp, evolved strong, flexible fibers that humans have used for a wide range of utilitarian purposes for the past 10,000 years.

Hemp arrived in the New World 53 years after Columbus first landed, but it is less clear when the smokable, intoxicating varieties of cannabis were imported. What we call marijuana today was brought to Brazil by the Portuguese and to Jamaica and other Caribbean islands by kidnapped Africans. The British also imported cannabis, primarily to pacify their slaves. It then arrived in the USA along four primary routes. Patent medicines from pharmaceutical companies containing cannabis extracts were popular through the mid- to late 1800s. Many Americans had their first puff of hash at the exotic Turkish Village in the 1893 Chicago World's Fair. Marijuana also arrived with sailors, Caribbean migrants filtering into New Orleans, and asylum seekers fleeing Mexico's violent revolution in 1910, primarily through El Paso. All the derogatory racial stereotypes that white Americans held regarding brown and Black people were quickly ascribed to marijuana as well. Its use by despised and feared minorities was alien to white American culture and reinforced prejudice against immigrants. Smokable cannabis and racism were intertwined from the very beginning, until white youth cracked the mold in the 1960s.

Before the Mexican-Spanish word "marihuana" first entered English usage, "cannabis" and variants of "hash" were the only terms used. Bristol Myers Squibb and Eli Lilly listed cannabis and cannabis extracts as ingredients in their medicines during the 1800s. The word "marijuana" was later popularized in racially derogatory stories about Mexican refugees. When Pancho Villa and his bandoliered men briefly invaded New Mexico in 1916, they openly flaunted their pot use as they sang creative verses of "La

Cucaracha" that included cockroaches smoking marijuana. But Pancho Villa's greater crime was when his support of land reform wrested 800,000 acres of timberland from newspaper magnate William Randolph Hearst during Mexico's uprising against foreign capitalist control. Hearst, who owned 8 million acres of Mexican land, used his media empire to strike back against the rebels by luridly sensationalizing both the Mexicans and marijuana.

In 1920, the USA joined Norway, Finland, and Russia in banning alcohol. This grand experiment of prohibition failed and was reversed in 1933, both because of the public's widespread disregard for the law and state governments' thirst for new tax revenue during the Great Depression. The Federal Bureau of Prohibition's assistant commissioner, Harry Anslinger, had become commissioner of the new Bureau of Narcotics in 1930. He initially had little interest in leading a campaign against what he saw as a mere weed; he insisted that cannabis was not a problem, did not harm people, and that "there is no more absurd fallacy" than the idea that it makes people violent. His mind changed with the deepening economic depression and end of alcohol prohibition. Fears that Mexican migrants might take scarce jobs intensified racial prejudice and combined with bureaucratic mission creep after alcohol was relegalized. William Randolph Hearst paved the way for Anslinger's conversion to anti-marijuana crusader by publishing a steady stream of stories about the evils of marijuana that reached 20 million daily readers during the 1930s. Hearst needed to sell newspapers, and racially charged descriptions of violent and sexual crimes caused by this killer weed sold very well.

Anslinger also hated the social threat he saw in jazz music. It was too wild, too frenzied, and too much the product of marijuana-smoking Black people from New Orleans. Jazz was becoming so popular that marijuana parlors featuring jazz music recordings were opened in

Harlem apartments during alcohol prohibition. Anslinger believed that white culture was being infected and degraded, and he used his position and racist rhetoric to place the blame on marijuana, even sensationalizing an axe murder without any evidence that marijuana was involved. Hearst baselessly claimed that three-quarters of all violent crimes were marijuana related, and Anslinger pointed directly to "Mexicans, Greeks, Turks, Filipinos, Spaniards, Latin Americans, and Negroes" as races enslaved to a drug that caused sexual degeneracy and insanity. Marijuana was consigned to being "other," existing outside the dominant white culture, just as Black and brown people were considered the "other." Anslinger's arguments for marijuana prohibition were not subtle. Even the word "marijuana" was charged with racial overtones.

The possession and sale of cannabis was effectively outlawed in 1937 by the Marihuana Tax Act. The act levied an outrageous tax on the stamps required for the sale and possession of marijuana, but the stamps were never truly made available. The plant and all those involved with it became outlaws. Despite his efforts, Anslinger failed to stop the spread of marijuana use and eventually became a laughingstock among Baby Boomers, who found marijuana very much to their liking. In the 1970s, theaters were routinely filled with stoned audiences mocking *Reefer Madness* and disparaging Anslinger's memory.

When marijuana use crept into white culture, first among beatniks in the 1950s and then exploding during the massive cultural shift of the 1960s to become a part of American life, it seemed to scrub racial slurs from the word "marijuana." The racial connotations associated with the word became less visible. Most white people are surprised to learn that the rate of marijuana use among white and Black people has been roughly the same for the past half century. In a cynical political move, President Nixon used his War on Drugs to criminalize marijuana-smoking

Vietnam War protesters and inner-city Black people. Again, marijuana and racial minorities were considered "other" and dangerous to America's interests. As the war on drug users intensified in the 1980s and fused with the country's craze for "getting tough on crime," America housed 25 percent of the world's prisoners, despite having only 5 percent of its total population. Racial undertones guided much of America's drug war. Despite the fact that only 13 percent of drug users are Black, reflecting their proportion of the overall population, Black people have been four times more likely to be arrested for marijuana possession and 13 times more likely to be sent to prison. Law enforcement agencies still systematically perceive an essential racial link between Black people and marijuana. The white majority has been largely unaware of this bias and, stoked by divisive politics, mounts too little an effort to reverse its perspective. There should be little wonder that dialog about cannabis remains dominated more by opinions about social values, with all their unconscious biases, than about objective, verifiable facts. Emotionally charged news reports and fear too often trump science in the political realm, and only increased science literacy about cannabis can swing the pendulum back toward rational discourse. As described in Chapter 1, science is an agreed-upon method for removing bias from what we think is fact. I will stick to the science throughout this book.

I will also stick to the word "cannabis," except for moments when slang seems more appropriate to the topic. Over time, the very meaning of "marijuana" has become confused. Even legal uses of the word refer variously to the whole cannabis plant, to parts of the plant that include both flowers and leaves, specifically only to dried flowers, and even to concentrated products from the plant. As a result of these inconsistently used terms and the history of racial denigration, the emerging industry increasingly uses the word "cannabis" rather than "marijuana." Even restricting "marijuana" to refer to smokable buds is gradually being replaced by the term "cannabis flowers."

Cannabis: What is This Plant?

The cannabis varieties of interest to us contain two families of chemical compounds: cannabinoids and terpenes. Cannabinoids are the most important because they produce the majority of the plant's psychoactive and medicinal properties. No other plant species on Earth contains these distinctive compounds. Terpenes, in contrast, are not at all unique in the plant world and are responsible for the characteristic smell of cannabis. Terpenes are found in a wide variety of plants, including pine trees, from which they are harvested and distilled into common turpentine, the volatile oil used in paints and liniments.

Over 100 different cannabinoid molecules have been identified in the cannabis plant, although only one is responsible for the bulk of the plant's psychoactive power. Known best by its initials, THC was first isolated in 1964 by a Bulgarian chemist who fled to Israel after World War II. The father of modern cannabinoid chemistry, Raphael Mechoulam had an addiction to research from which he did not want to be cured. Searching for an important topic to establish his career, Mechoulam saw a prime opportunity in the mystery of how cannabis works. He decided to attempt to isolate its essential, mind-altering ingredient. In order to get enough raw material for his research, Mechoulam asked his supervisor to vouch for him with an old army buddy up the road in Tel Aviv's police headquarters. The police offered 11 lb (5 kg) of hash, the concentrated resinous goo secreted by cannabis flowers, if Mechoulam would pick it up personally. Without access to a car, Mechoulam took a bus to Tel Aviv. On the ride back to his laboratory, the other passengers wondered about the

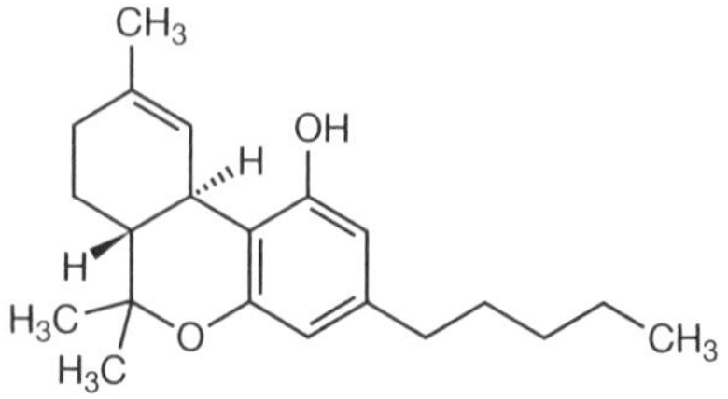

Figure 2.2 Molecular structure of Δ^9-tetrahydrocannabinol (THC).

intense odor coming from his bag. Mechoulam has often expressed appreciation for working in a small country where bureaucratic red tape can be sliced through so easily.

Mechoulam's diverse research team of Israelis, Palestinians, an American, a Czech, Jews, Muslims, and Christians were the first to purify THC and determine its molecular structure (Figure 2.2). In a three-step process, his team confirmed that this single molecule produces most of the mind-altering effects of cannabis. First, monkeys given THC behaved like they do when given whole-cannabis extracts. Second, they found that cannabis with THC removed had no effect. And third, Mechoulam invited some members of his research team to experience the effects of pure THC. Those given a placebo were unaffected, while those administered THC reported feeling strange, giggly, or anxious. Research team members who had pre-viously used cannabis recognized and verified that THC felt similar.

Mechoulam tells a revealing anecdote about his efforts to get the US National Institute on Drug Abuse (NIDA) to fund his grant application for THC research. NIDA rejected the grant request because they felt marijuana use was not a significant issue in the USA. When the head of NIDA heard Mechoulam had purified THC, he flew to Israel to discuss the discovery. Apparently, the importance of adolescent cannabis use had taken a higher priority after an influential senator contacted NIDA for information when he caught his son smoking pot. The NIDA Director returned to the USA with 10 grams of pure THC in his pocket, and Mechoulam has received NIDA funding ever since without experiencing any interference from the US government.

Cannabis contains many compounds similar to the structure of THC with little or no known medical or recreational importance. The one exception is cannabidiol, more commonly known as CBD. While CBD alone has only a slight anti-anxiety effect, it has many important, proven medicinal properties. Both the promise and hype surrounding CBD will be examined more closely in Chapter 9.

The amounts of THC and CBD in every strain of cannabis are inversely related to each other; this means that a plant with high THC has low CBD, and vice versa. This inverse relationship impacts the experience and safety of cannabis and cannabis products, and can be illustrated by a farmer whose cow produces one pail of milk a day. The farmer can make either butter or cheese from the pail of milk. The more butter the farmer makes, the less cheese can be made from the milk left in the pail. The more cheese the farmer makes, the less butter will be possible.

Both THC and CBD are made from the same finite amount of the cannabinoid named CBG (cannabigerol). Two enzymes compete to synthesize THC and CBD from the limited pail of CBG available. Strains of cannabis differ in the amount of these two enzymes. Strains with a high amount of the THC-synthesizing enzyme produce buds with the most psychoactivity but the least CBD. While clever crossbreeding has produced cannabis strains with an increasingly large pail of CBG, leading to larger amounts of both THC and CBD, an inverse ratio between the two continues to be the rule. The negative impact of a high THC:CBD ratio on the safety of cannabis will be discussed in later chapters.

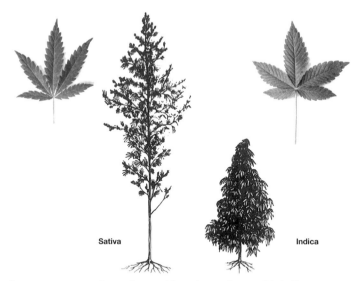

Sativa   Indica

Figure 2.3 Comparison of *Cannabis sativa* and *Cannabis indica*.

A lot of attention has been paid to the differences between the two major species of cannabis, *Cannabis sativa* and *Cannabis indica*, but this has become a futile and confusing exercise. When cannabis was left to evolve in nature, sativa plants grew 20 ft (6 m) tall with long, narrow leaves that are a lighter shade of green. Indica plants have broader leaves and are much shorter and stockier. With a maximum height of only 6 ft (1.8 m) and flowering in roughly half the time of sativa, indica plants are preferred for growing indoors (Figure 2.3). These two species are generally seen as having different psychoactive profiles. Indica is described as having a deeply relaxing effect called a "body high," while sativa is energizing, stimulating, and more of a "mental high."

However, the distinction between these two species has become confusing because most cannabis sold today is a hybrid of the two. Horticulturists continue breeding novel hybrids to accelerate cannabis evolution and satisfy human desire, an idea nicely developed by Michael Pollan in his book, *The Botany of Desire*. The first phase of cannabis evolution was propelled by changes in climate and predators. Cannabis is now in its second phase of evolution, guided by human desire for intoxication and medicinal benefits. Understanding the basic effects of THC and CBD on the body and brain is more relevant than drawing distinctions between changing hybrid brands.

In 1968, the US government contracted with the Department of Pharmaceutical Sciences at the University of Mississippi to grow marijuana that could be standardized for research. Mahmoud ElSohly, an Egyptian postdoctoral student, joined the Marijuana Project in 1975 and has been its Director since 1981; he expanded the farm to 12 heavily secured acres and began analyzing marijuana seized across the country. ElSohly's PhD in the pharmacology of natural products had taken him in a unique direction – he was the only legal cannabis grower in the USA. He appreciates the incongruity of his career path and says that his twin daughters often cheekily answered teachers' questions about what their father did by saying, "He grows marijuana," only later adding that he was a professor at the University of Mississippi.

ElSohly says we should think of the intense hybridization of indica and sativa as creating three types of marijuana plants: those with high levels of THC and low CBD, those with equal amounts of each, and those with low THC and high CBD. He notes that in the 1980s, the THC:CBD ratio of most marijuana was 10:1 or 15:1. In 2017, that ratio jumped 100-fold, leaving THC's impact largely unmodified by CBD's balancing effects (discussed further in Chapter 3). High-dose THC with minimal CBD increases the incidence of negative side effects.

Cannabis strains without THC and only minimal CBD have long been cultivated for their versatile fibers.

Generally called hemp, the earliest evidence of its use occurred 10,000 years ago in China, woven into cords found with pottery. Hemp fiber contributed to the rope and canvas sails that helped seafaring nations explore the world. The very word "canvas" comes from cannabis. Jamestown settlers carried hemp to Virginia in 1611, and its cultivation quickly spread through the American colonies, as evidenced by mentions of the hemp crop at Mount Vernon in George Washington's diary. Over the centuries, hemp has been used to produce everything from rope and sails to paper, clothing, biodegradable plastics, paint, insulation, biofuel, and animal feed. While our concerns focus on those strains of cannabis that produce resin laden with THC, some attention will be given to hemp as a source of CBD in Chapter 9.

The word "marijuana" refers specifically to the dried flower buds of female cannabis plants containing psychoactive and medicinal properties (i.e. THC and/or CBD). Male plants do not contain recreational or medicinal cannabinoids, but they do provide the pollen necessary for female flowers to produce seeds. Before seeds are produced, female plants secrete sticky resin that contains the active cannabinoids that humans desire. Scientists are still not sure why cannabis plants secrete this resin, but it can only be assumed that this unique evolutionary development confers some survival advantage to cannabis. As the species developed well before humans evolved, its psychoactive properties were not developed to attract our attention. Was it a defense against external threats, like harmful microbes, insects, or plant eaters? Did it protect the plant from environmental dangers, like the cold, dehydrating wind, drought, or ultraviolet radiation at the high elevation where cannabis evolved? Was it to attract pollinating insects and seed-spreading animals? After all, many flowers attract bees by secreting small amounts of caffeine in their nectar.

If male plants are weeded out before they can pollinate females, more resin is produced, but no seeds. "Sinsemilla," from the Spanish for "without seeds," is highly potent marijuana from unpollinated female plants, a gardening technique used to increase marijuana's strength and value. The THC content of marijuana has risen steadily over the years, from 3 percent during the 1960s to an average in the high teens available in dispensaries today. The highest-documented THC content is a strain named Future, containing an astounding 37 percent THC. However, claims that today's pot is a new drug are not technically true. Just as the alcohol molecule found in high-proof liquor is no different from that found in beer, the THC in today's marijuana is no newer than the THC from the 1960s. However, it does contain higher concentrations of THC, so the speed with which modern marijuana impacts the brain and the intensity of impact are greater, thereby increasing the pleasure, potential medical value, and negative side effects.

Cannabis Products

Recent developments in manufacturing techniques that extract the cannabinoid molecules found in cannabis flower have resulted in a variety of new products for eating, vaping, and other forms of consumption.

Attitudes toward psychoactive cannabis products have swung wildly throughout history. During the last half of the 1800s, before the word marijuana entered the English language, cannabis extracts were included in many over-the-counter patent medicines. The extent of America's comfort with cannabis is charmingly illustrated by the Gunjah Wallah Company's maple-sugar "hasheesh candy," which was one of America's most popular treats from 1860 to 1900. For ease of shopping, Sears, Roebuck and Co. offered the candy through their mail-order catalog, calling it a "most pleasurable and harmless stimulant – Cures Nervousness, Weakness, Melancholy, &c. Inspires all classes with new life and energy. A complete mental and physical invigorator."

Colorado dispensaries report that cannabis flower initially comprised 67 percent of sales in 2014. Within 5 years, flower sales fell to 44 percent, replaced by manufactured cannabis products, including edibles (e.g. cookies, brownies, and gummy bears), beverages (sodas, teas, shots), and vaporizers similar to e-cigarettes. THC vaping cartridges (called e-juice) are available in bubble gum, banana nut bread, and cotton candy flavors, which are advertised as opening up exciting new ways to consume cannabis. Vaping is especially effective at swiftly producing very high THC levels in the blood.

Cannabis oil waxes are an even more powerful way to ingest THC quickly. Wax is manufactured through a dangerous process of extracting THC from cannabis flowers with highly flammable butane. Once butane hash oil (BHO) is extracted, the waxy product needs to be purified by heating it to evaporate the butane. The end product, variously called shatter, budder, or wax, depending on its appearance, contains up to 90 percent THC. Videos on YouTube illustrate how to produce wax at home, but because butane is extremely explosive, these techniques are not safe in the hands of amateurs. Wax is consumed by dabbing, a method that requires a heated rig to instantaneously vaporize the wax for inhaling. The resulting high is the quickest and most intense that cannabis offers, as THC oil cannot be injected intravenously because it does not dissolve in water. Dabbing's impact can be intense enough to cause hallucinations and is increasing in popularity.

Conclusion

The bud regally sitting on purple velvet that Martin offered me had come a long way from the scrubby cannabis plants that first appeared on the high Tibetan plateau almost 30 million years ago. Carried around the world by travelers, migrants, merchants, healers, and mystics, and lovingly crossbred and nurtured, this dry bud held secrets explored by both scientists and cannabis connoisseurs. As I looked at this mystical, brown bud, I thought of the brain inside my skull that was pondering what makes cannabis so powerfully intriguing. I knew that the secrets of cannabis lay as much in what our brains do with the bud's chemistry as they do in the plant itself. Botany is only one part of the story.

Unless you understand how the chemistry and physiology of your brain interacts with cannabis, you will never fully appreciate its power or know how to use it safely. *Cannabis affects brain function, and is therefore mind-altering, only because the brain is wired to respond to THC and CBD.*

There is much more to learn about the cannabis plant, especially if you are interested in botany or want to grow it yourself. Bookstores and online retailers offer a wide variety of excellent books devoted to cannabis cultivation, including the use of hydroponics and specialized grow lights, but no amount of botanical knowledge will help you understand how cannabis works, either recreationally or medicinally. For that story, we turn to a brief description of how brain cells communicate with each other, and then to an explanation of the brain's own natural THC-like chemistry, to explore how marijuana works.

3 THE BRAIN AND ITS NATURAL CANNABINOID CHEMISTRY

Sarah was 15 and already devoted to cannabis, despite the legal difficulties she faced from being caught smoking a joint in the school bathroom. I had no hope of convincing her that the risks she ran were serious, so I took a different approach, hoping to intrigue her into learning more about weed. I asked what she liked most about being high.

"It chills me out," she said. When I asked her to elaborate, she explained how it relaxed her, how it quieted her monkey mind and constant worrying. She had been anxious for as long as she could remember. As there had been no significant traumas in her life, I assumed she was suffering from a primary anxiety disorder. She had been born with the temperament of a mouse, meaning a tense and restless tendency to be constantly ready for danger and looking for it everywhere. She was attracted to cannabis because it eased the symptoms of her anxiety disorder.

"What do you know about how cannabis works?" I asked. She had no idea and admitted that she had never really thought about it. I began explaining how cannabis controlled the anxiety caused by excess activity in a part of her brain, using some of the information contained in this chapter. Because I paid attention to the specific ways in which cannabis benefited her, she listened and became interested in what I told her about her brain.

This chapter braids together several scientific threads to build a foundation for understanding how the brain is wired to respond to cannabis. Understanding this wiring is crucial for understanding how cannabis works. The language is as plain and the explanations as simple as possible, given the complexity of the human brain. If you can bear some geekiness along the way, you will be rewarded with a firm grasp of the brain's marvelous mechanics and its response to cannabis. You will also learn basic concepts about the brain that are needed to understand why there are limits to how frequently cannabis can safely be used, limits that are inherent in how the brain interacts with THC.

Neuroscience 101: Communication Between Nerve Cells

Our brain is the most complex organization of matter in the universe. Personally, I subscribe to what I call the "firefly" model of the brain. Also known as lightning bugs, fireflies are beetles that use short bursts of light to attract each other during mating season. Some fireflies can synchronize their flashing, a feat that is of relevance to this discussion. In late May to mid-June, synchronized flashing can be seen in Great Smoky Mountains National Park, sometimes in waves across mountainsides. An Australian species has been known to congregate on a single bush and flash on and off like a Christmas light display. Although these fireflies are separate animals, they are connected by the sending and receiving of light signals.

The brain is made up of nerve cells, called neurons. The average human brain weighs 3 lb (1.3 kg) and contains a staggering 90 billion neurons, all tangled and highly interconnected. Each neuron is essentially a single-celled animal, similar to an amoeba and just as capable of living independently in a Petri dish. Despite this fact, nerve cells achieve an astonishing degree of collaboration in their activity, executing rhythmic pulses seen as brain waves on an electroencephalogram (EEG) and a level of coordination that far surpasses the swirling flight of a group of starlings. Healthy neurons continue to fire as long as we live. Like fireflies, neurons collaborate and achieve synchrony by sending and receiving signals. In the brain, these signals are small bursts of chemicals transmitted between neurons, and are therefore called neurotransmitters.

Some neurons stretch from the base of our spine to the end of our toes, more than 3 ft (0.9 m) in very tall people. This extraordinary length is accomplished by an extension from each neuron cell body called an axon, which is like a wire that allows neurons to reach out to one another, as well as to connect with muscles and other parts of the body. When many axons run together through the body, we call them nerves. When bundles of axons run through the brain, they are called nerve tracts and constitute the brain's white matter. In contrast, gray matter is made of nerve cell bodies. It is found in the cortex that lines the surface of the brain and in collections of nerve cell bodies below the surface. Cannabis affects both gray and white matter, although in different ways. The acute effects of ingesting cannabis result from its impact on gray matter, while the impact on white matter happens over time with regular use.

The basic structure of neurons is illustrated schematically in Figure 3.1. Neurons are unique among the body's cells because of their specialized ability to communicate with each other and to form extraordinarily complex networks. Each neuron's axon forms close connections with the cell body of as many as 10,000 other neurons. These connections are made on short extensions called dendrites. Axons sometimes take circuitous routes as long as 12 in (30 cm) to connect neuron cell bodies on the two sides of the brain. Connections between neurons are extremely close, but neurons do not quite touch. The minute gap

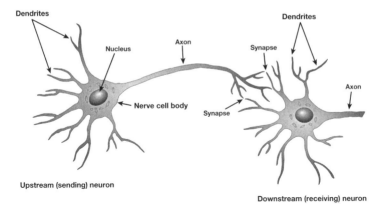

Figure 3.1 Schematic of the structure of neurons.

between neurons is called a synapse, a term from the Greek word *synapsis*, meaning "joined together." There are a nearly inconceivable number of synapses in the human brain – roughly five times as many as there are stars in the Milky Way galaxy!

Neurons send chemical messengers across synapses to either increase or inhibit the activity of the next neuron. The experience of chemical messaging is actually familiar to all of us. If you were blindfolded and someone held a freshly cut lemon up to your nose, most people would be immediately able to sense and identify the fragrant molecules stimulating the nerves in their nose. Differentiating between lemon, lime, pepper, onion, cloves, cinnamon, and garlic, for example, is quite simple. The 40 million smell receptors in our nose can detect a trillion different odors. Similar chemical signaling constantly takes place throughout the brain, not as fast as light between fireflies or data through a computer, but with a far richer variety of chemical messengers and with parallel processing on a grand scale.

People often say that neurons pass information through the brain; this is both correct and incorrect. Neurons only pass signals, like the ones and zeros in binary code, or like the dots and dashes of Morse code. Information does not lie in each dot or dash, but rather in the *pattern* of dots and dashes. A telegrapher receiving a random mix of dots and dashes receives no information. However, three dots followed by three dashes and again by three dots will cause a telegrapher to jump into action to respond to a sinking ship's SOS. Neurons receive information by interpreting the pattern of chemical messengers simultaneously received from as many as 10,000 synapses, and their cumulative effect will be transmitted on to another 10,000 distant neurons. It seems beyond our capacity to make sense of such complexity, but human brains routinely coordinate this complex activity effectively enough to hunt for prey or groceries, hit home runs, and read books. Our brains do not have to understand how they work in order to carry out the work for which they are designed.

Each neuron uses only one of several known chemical neurotransmitters. Dopamine, serotonin, and endorphins are three commonly known neurotransmitters, but over 40 have been identified. Each neuron synthesizes its particular neurotransmitter from DNA instructions contained in the cell body's nucleus. The neurotransmitter molecules are then transported through the axon to be stored near synapses. When an electrical impulse firing down the axon at up to 275 miles (442 km) per hour reaches the axon's tip, neurotransmitter is released into the synapse and almost instantaneously arrives at the outer membrane of the downstream neuron. However, when researching how marijuana works, scientists discovered that this is only half of the story.

Neurons, like all cells in the body, are filled with water and bathed in extracellular fluid outside the cell. The only thing dividing the watery compartment inside the cell from the outside is a thin, fatty membrane, like the film of a soap bubble. As oil and water do not mix, fatty cell membranes maintain the integrity of the neuron's internal environment while keeping the machinery inside the cell from drifting off. Like our skin, which keeps us from soaking up water when we swim or bathe and yet permits perspiration to leave the body when we are too warm, cell membranes actively regulate what comes in and goes out of cells. Cell membranes permit ions, such as sodium, potassium, chloride, and calcium, to exist in different concentrations on the outside and inside of the cell. Like a tiny battery, this difference in ion concentration creates a slight electrical gradient across the membrane. When a neuron fires, a quick disturbance in this gradient travels like a wave down the axon to release neurotransmitter in the synapses.

On the downstream side of synapses, chemical receptors sit astride neuronal membranes, as seen in Figure 3.2, with one side of the receptor sticking out of the cell and the opposite side sticking into the cell. Normally locked, receptors do not permit anything to enter or leave the cell. When a neurotransmitter enters a receptor for which it is uniquely designed, like a key entering a lock, the receptor changes shape to allow a brief rush of ions to enter, either exciting or inhibiting the neuron's activity. The neurotransmitter is quickly metabolized by enzymes designed to limit the length of its action on the receptor, while other specialized molecules sweep up extra neurotransmitter and transport it back into the axon terminal. Voila! Chemical signaling, like a well-oiled machine. This is how the brain works, through almost infinitely complex networks of synaptic connections, all simultaneously processing incomprehensible numbers of signals. That it works at all is amazing. That it is capable of coordinating movement of a person's body is staggering. That it can move a person's hand to pick up a quill to create *Hamlet*, coining several new words in a play that moves us emotionally over 400 years later, is beyond my powers of comprehension. I can only stand in awe.

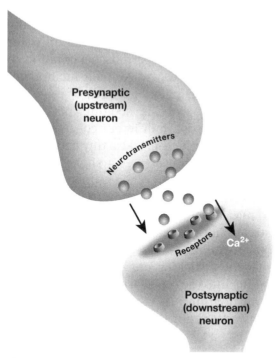

Figure 3.2 A typical neurotransmitter crossing a synapse.

How all this brain activity, born of constantly fluctuating alchemical communication among billions of single-celled animals, gives rise to our conscious experience is beyond even the world's best neuroscientists and philosophers to explain. Early in my career, I observed patients with brain death from strokes and drug overdoses lying senseless. Consciousness clearly arises from brain activity. As we shall soon see, when THC alters brain activity, the mind and conscious experience are also altered.

Sarah listened politely to my description of how her brain works through chemical communication among nerve cells, and only responded with interest to the idea of nerves "smelling" each other. That was enough. When

I later explained how the brain's response to cannabis eventually becomes blunted, she compared this to how her mother no longer smelled her stale cigarette smoke that filled her home.

Neuroscience 102: The Brain's Natural Cannabinoids

Since Raphael Mechoulam isolated THC in 1964, research has taught us precisely how cannabis alters the chemical balance and activity in the brain. Our experience of this altered activity is called "getting high" when voluntarily sought, a medical benefit, or a "side effect" when unpleasant.

After THC was purified and its molecular structure determined, the race was on to discover how THC interacts with the brain. In 1988, scientists announced the monumental discovery of a receptor in the brain that is activated by THC. We soon learned that there are two different cannabinoid receptors: CB1, found primarily in the brain, and CB2, found in the rest of the body. Most researchers assumed that the existence of receptors that can be unlocked by cannabis molecules meant a natural THC-like neurotransmitter must also be present. After all, it is unlikely that our brains possess a cannabinoid receptor solely for getting high, especially when researchers discovered that the cannabinoid receptor can be found in virtually all animals, except insects, and is the most common receptor in the human brain. The most likely explanation was that cannabinoid receptors play a natural function in the brain by responding to an as-yet-undiscovered cannabinoid-like neurotransmitter. This prospect captured Sarah's interest and she sat up straighter.

It took only 4 years for Mechoulam's laboratory to discover the first of our brain's natural cannabinoid neurotransmitters. During that time, researchers at the National

Institutes of Health (NIH) added important information to the cascade of new discoveries about cannabinoid receptors. As NIH scientists mapped the location of CB1 receptors, they immediately saw a correspondence between several characteristics of being high and the parts of the brain where CB1 receptors are most densely concentrated. For example, the part of the brain where short-term memory forms is heavily packed with CB1 receptors. This was immediately assumed to be related to the short-term memory loss often experienced when high. Heavy concentrations of CB1 receptors in motor and emotional areas of the brain correlate with physical relaxation, sometimes to the point of what has been dubbed "couch lock," and the quelling of anxiety experienced with cannabis use. Also, virtually no CB1 receptors were seen in the brain stem, where breathing reflexes are found. This explains why cannabis never causes the type of death seen in opiate overdoses. Opiate receptors are plentiful in the brain stem, where their activation slows, and eventually stops, breathing.

While the NIH was cloning and mapping the location of CB1 receptors, Mechoulam's research team was working to isolate and identify a THC-like neurotransmitter native to the brain. By 1992, they had collected and purified 0.000021 oz (0.6 mg) of a natural brain chemical that bound to CB1 receptors from 10 lb (4.5 kg) of pig brains. A member of Mechoulam's team was studying Sanskrit at the time and suggested the name "anandamide," meaning "supreme joy or bliss," as a way of expressing the feeling of exquisite joy that comes with being the first to make a significant scientific discovery. Sarah thought there might have been other reasons for naming our brain's natural cannabinoid chemical "supreme joy."

Scientists who discovered the brain's natural opiate compounds had already established a tradition for naming a new class of neurotransmitters that are imitated by plants. These earlier researchers had begun with the poppy plant, which produces a sticky resin (opium) with strong psychoactive properties. Just as THC was found to be the active ingredient in cannabis resin, morphine was identified as the active ingredient in opium. After opiate receptors were discovered in the brain, scientists searched for a natural, morphine-like neurotransmitter. When they found it, they collapsed two words to name it. The first word, endogenous, meaning "having an internal origin," was combined with morphine to create the word endorphin. Consequently, Mechoulam classified his purified endogenous cannabinoid neurotransmitter, anandamide, as an "endocannabinoid." This remains the name for a class of now over a dozen related endogenous cannabinoid neurotransmitters.

Mechoulam noticed a resemblance between the structure of anandamide and a fatty building block common to all cell membranes called arachidonic acid. It was soon established that anandamide is synthesized on demand from arachidonic acid at the synapse itself, unlike other neurotransmitters that have to be transported down axons to synapses after being synthesized in the neuron cell body. With the discovery of CB1 receptors, anandamide, and the unexpected location of anandamide's synthesis, questions arose about how this neurochemical system fitted into the brain's structure and function. The answer changed some of our basic understanding of how the brain works. When a Hungarian scientist, István Katona, discovered the unique location of CB1 receptors, the function of our endogenous cannabinoid (or endocannabinoid) system (ECS) rapidly fell into place.

The basic structure and function of our brain's ECS can be described in one paragraph. When any neurotransmitter is released, it travels across the synapse and binds to its unique receptor. This sets several things in motion. The activated receptor allows an influx of ions into the

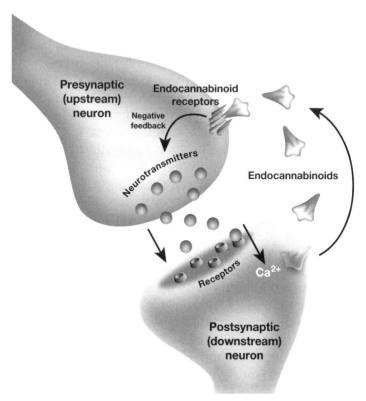

Figure 3.3 The endocannabinoid system's negative-feedback system.

downstream neuron, which either excites or inhibits the neuron's activity. At the same time, this influx of ions stimulates synthesis of anandamide from arachidonic acid molecules in the downstream neuron's cell membrane. Once synthesized, anandamide returns across the synapse to bind with CB1 receptors on the upstream neuron, causing an influx of ions there. This influx of ions acts as a negative feedback on the upstream neuron's release of neurotransmitter (Figure 3.3).

The ECS is a negative-feedback system designed to maintain chemical balance among all the other brain neurotransmitters. The brain's natural cannabinoid system is the master regulator of brain chemistry. We discovered this system, so fundamentally important to proper brain function and mental/emotional well-being, only because we were trying to understand how cannabis works. When neurons become more active, the increased amount of neurotransmitter they release stimulates more endocannabinoid synthesis by downstream neurons, which then causes the upstream neurons to release less neurotransmitter each time they fire. The frequency of neurotransmitter release is not changed, but the amount of neurotransmitter released with each firing is reduced. This prevents receptors from being overwhelmed by too much stimulation. Then, when upstream neurons lower their firing rate, the amount of negative feedback also decreases. The frequency of firing is less now, but a larger amount of neurotransmitter is released with each firing. The ECS regulates every other neurotransmitter system to keep the brain chemically balanced. Figure 3.3 traces the entire negative-feedback loop, from upstream to downstream neuron and back again.

The ECS is always active, its tone increasing or decreasing in response to changing levels of upstream neuronal activity. The ECS is a homeostatic system designed to maintain brain chemistry stability. A healthy brain, and therefore a healthy mind, depends on a properly functioning ECS.

Neuroscience 103: THC Interactions with the Brain

In Figure 3.4, you'll see two molecular structures. On the left is the three-dimensional molecular structure of anandamide, and on the right is the structure of THC.

There are minor differences between the shapes of anandamide and THC, but not enough to prevent THC from

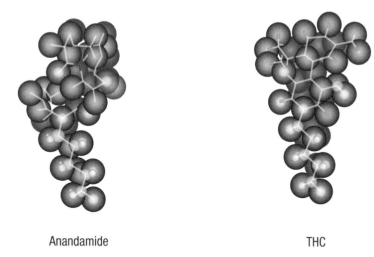

Anandamide   THC

Figure 3.4 Similarity of the molecular structure of anandamide and THC.

fitting into cannabinoid receptors. *THC interacts with the brain by mimicking natural endocannabinoid neurotransmitters.* As a result, THC activates CB1 receptors and simultaneously initiates negative feedback on upstream neurons in a wide range of neurotransmitter systems throughout the brain. This mimicry has a multitude of consequences that will be explored in the rest of this and following chapters.

THC's activation of CB1 receptors throughout the brain is not a homeostatic process. The negative feedback resulting from THC is not in reaction to increased upstream neuronal activity but rather is a blanket activation of all CB1 receptors that disrupts the normal balance among all the neurotransmitter systems. The result is harder to calculate than it is to observe and experience. While scientists study the impact of THC on those experiencing it, their observations provide very different information when compared with the direct, subjective experience of being high. We need to look closely at both perspectives.

Widespread negative feedback on multiple neurotransmitter systems does not necessarily mean a total reduction of brain activity. Some brain functions are diminished: memory, anxiety, and spontaneous movement, for example. Other functions are stimulated: hunger, sensory experience, and the sense of novelty. Complicating matters even further, different strains of cannabis produce different profiles of inhibition and excitement due to differences in their relative amounts of THC and CBD. Employees of your local cannabis dispensary (called budistas, a word borrowed from baristas, or budtenders, borrowed from bartenders) will offer their opinions on the wide range of variable effects found in the different varieties they sell.

Most importantly, THC does not precisely mimic our endocannabinoids. Instead, when THC binds to CB1 receptors in the brain and CB2 receptors in the body, it activates a response that is both far stronger and longer than our natural endocannabinoids. This fact is of paramount importance for understanding cannabis, both its immediate effects (Chapter 4) and why its use has limits imposed by the brain's resistance to these effects (Chapter 10). The speed and length of THC's impact depends on the dose and mode of delivery. Dabbing highly concentrated hash oil can be felt almost immediately and can last up to 3 hours. Inhaling smoked cannabis flower can be felt within 2–10 minutes and lasts 4–8 hours. Edibles (cannabis-infused food products) can take 2 hours to have an effect but this effect can last for 12–24 hours. The slow onset of THC edibles is responsible for inexperienced or impatient users repeating a dose too quickly and ultimately overdosing to an uncomfortable degree. As a result, cannabis tourists flying out of Denver's airport frequently realize too late that their edibles are still illegal back home and inadvertently overdose rather than throw their souvenirs in the trash. By the time their flight is ready to board, they have become so paranoid and panicked that they are deemed "too high to fly" and have to be diverted to a local emergency room.

The bottom line is that THC is not naturally found in the body and does not accurately mimic anandamide or other endocannabinoids. It behaves more like a long-acting cannabinoid on steroids, overloading cannabinoid receptors throughout the entire brain and body. This global, unnaturally strong activation of cannabinoid receptors has little immediate medical danger, except perhaps the risk of a moderate increase in heart rate in someone with significant pre-existing heart disease. Many people enjoy the mind-altering experience of THC's temporary overactivation of their entire ECS, much as many average citizens enjoy the temporary global suppression of neuronal activity following a couple of alcoholic drinks. As long as neither is repeated often enough to modify brain function between each use, this should probably be seen as a lifestyle choice. Whether or not you choose to partake in cannabis from time to time, your choice is unlikely to be of much medical concern.

Conclusion

While the brain is forced to function differently when our ECS is pushed far beyond its normal balance, THC does not make the brain do anything it is not designed to do. Endocannabinoid receptors are designed to produce negative feedback on upstream neurons, which is also what THC makes them do, although to an unnatural degree. Alcohol, in contrast, disrupts the physical structure of cell membranes, among its many effects, causing cell membranes to become more porous. Over time, alcohol can destroy enough brain cells to cause profound dementia, something cannabis has never been shown to cause.

Most people who use cannabis are naturally curious about how THC produces the experiences they enjoy when high, even though they may have little interest in what science says about the risks of using. Sarah listened to me long enough to learn that her brain has a natural THC-like chemistry. She thought that was cool. She also learned that her anxiety comes from excess activity in the part of her brain that cannabis suppresses. While she did not listen to my explanation that quelling her anxiety with cannabis can paradoxically increase anxiety when the high wears off, she had at least begun to think about how she was managing her brain with the pot. Sarah especially liked thinking of cannabis as being like her natural cannabinoids on powerful steroids, although it gave her pause when I reminded her of the toll steroids eventually take on the body. She agreed to see me again to talk more about what she liked about getting high, and I took this as another possible opportunity to increase her interest in what cannabis does in the brain.

Using THC to activate our brain's ECS beyond its normal physiological limits does not produce the same experience for everyone because personalities and brains differ. The circumstances under which cannabis is taken differ. Cannabis strains also differ. But if we listen to what people who use cannabis recreationally say about their experience, there is a great deal of overlap. Chapter 4 takes the reader inside this experience and then analyzes the specific changes in brain function that give rise to different aspects of the typical cannabis user's high.

4 THE PLANT'S IMPACT ON THE BRAIN AND EXPERIENCE

Tom thoroughly enjoyed introducing his friends to cannabis. He was careful. You had to be careful in 1967 in central Ohio. He was careful about where he bought his marijuana, relying on an old high-school friend who grew his own rather than his new friends at Ohio State University who were eager to sell him their wares. He was careful to groom his stash, diligently picking out all the seeds and stems. And he was very careful to wait for his friends to express curiosity before beginning a conversation about pot.

Tom took marijuana's mystique and power seriously. He had distrusted authority throughout high school, resisting teachers' dominance often to his own detriment. He suffered no fools, and when he saw rigidity or foolishness in older adults, he was quick to tell them so. As soon as he got to college, Tom seized on the first opportunity he had to try marijuana. He had never believed the scare tactics about the plant, and it took only a few puffs to confirm that no one over the age of 30 deserved his trust. He wanted his friends to experience what he had learned about the marvels of being high.

The thing I admired most about Tom was his understanding of the power of cannabis. He was serious about preparing people before they tried marijuana for the first time, discussing their expectations and fears to be sure he could keep them safe. He encouraged them to think carefully about their motivations and asked them to weigh their decision for a few days. Then he provided the safest environment he could to make it a quality experience. Tom took his role of cannabis guide seriously.

Set and Setting

When Napoleon's army returned from their conquest of Egypt, soldiers brought back more than memories; they also brought hash to France. By the mid-1840s, the oily cannabis extract had become all the rage among intellectuals and artists in Paris. The Club des Haschischins, a group of Parisian intellectuals who would meet to consume hashish, included such illustrious authors as Victor Hugo, Honoré de Balzac, Alexandre Dumas, and Charles Baudelaire. Members of the club quickly learned that hash intoxication made them very susceptible to both the environment in which it was taken (the *setting*) and to the user's mood and expectations (the mindset, or *set*). Baudelaire cautioned, "Any grief, anxiety, or thoughts of duty that may call on your will and attention at certain moments will cut like a death-knell right through your intoxication, and poison all your pleasure." He wrote that a positive experience is more likely "if you find yourself in the right environment, such as a picturesque landscape or an apartment that has been decorated artistically, and if you can also hope for a little music."

The concepts of set and setting have become central to our thinking about the experience of being under the influence of any psychoactive drug. If cannabis is first experienced furtively, reluctantly, or while fearful of punishment, the experience is more likely to be negative, even panicky and paranoid. If the first experience is sought out of curiosity, guided by a trusted friend, and in safe, comfortable surroundings, the experience is far more likely to be positive. This makes it difficult to characterize the drug's effect, as so much of the experience is influenced by the user's expectations and circumstances. Baudelaire noted that the same individual can have radically different experiences depending on his or her internal state (rested and relaxed, or tired and tense) and external surroundings (among many strangers or with a small group of friends).

The term "set and setting" was coined in 1964 by Timothy Leary, the Harvard professor turned LSD guru. Scientists generally accept that the effects of drugs such as cannabis and the major psychedelics are highly dependent on your mindset (personality, preparation, expectations) and the physical, social, and cultural environment in which the drug is experienced. Set and setting. Keep these factors firmly in mind as you read the following description of my personal introduction to cannabis.

A First Experience with Cannabis

My curiosity about marijuana began more than 50 years ago. I first met Mary Jane on a cool, summer evening in Columbus, Ohio, where I was completing my pre-med requirements. I had just graduated from a small, liberal arts college 20 miles up the road and years behind the cultural shifts taking place at Ohio State University. It was 1967, and America was barreling toward worsening violence in Vietnam, angrier war protests, more race turmoil, political assassinations, and a police riot in Chicago. My close friend since high school, Tom, had marinated in the burgeoning radicalism at OSU and offered me the chance to sample a different world from the corn fields that had surrounded me for the past 4 years. Was I curious? I was.

A skilled guide, Tom reassured me by staying straight, having ice water ready when the harsh smoke rasped my throat, and sitting me in front of his comforting fireplace. When he asked why I had been staring so intently at the flames, I was suddenly called back to his apartment, surprised that only 15 minutes had passed during the deeply relaxed reverie I had enjoyed. I expounded in awe that I had been watching the oxygen atoms combine with carbon in the flame. When their outer electron shells merged, they released energy – heat and light – as the orange vapors from the burning logs flickered and danced. It was chemistry and beauty fused together. "It's truly beautiful," I said earnestly.

"You've had enough," Tom confirmed with a smile, and then encouraged me to lie back and close my eyes.

The first thing I noticed after settling back was the music. It took on a new physical quality as my body resonated with individual notes. The stereophonic separation of instruments emphasized the room's three-dimensional volume. I realized that the music was simply vibrations in air pressure against my eardrums transmitted by sensory nerve impulses to my brain. The only place the *experience* of sound occurred was in my consciousness, in the brain activity these impulses evoked. If a tree fell in the forest and no sentient being was present to experience it, there was no sound, only concussive waves of pressure traveling through the air. When I understood that the sound of music existed only inside my skull, the most remarkable thing occurred: I experienced my head expand to fill the room. The "sound" within my brain was being hurled out into the room like a ventriloquist's voice into the mouth of a dummy. I was experiencing my brain's internal response to the music being projected out into the room, where stereo speakers were pumping guitar and drum vibrations against the air. I was already enthralled by marijuana.

As the fantastic images began to fade, I reviewed them several times to commit the experience to memory, and then focused on how relaxed and immobile my body felt. I thought of moving but continued to lie still. I wondered how it was possible for a conscious decision to cause the whole complex of matter comprising my body to transport through space to a new position in the universe, that is, to sit up. Mind over matter? I continued lying motionless, unmotivated to attempt movement but wondering what would happen if I did choose to move.

Tom returned and asked if anyone wanted a warm brownie, baked from a box without any pot added. I sat up immediately without having to plan how to accomplish the feat. "But first," he instructed, "open up." He popped a single SweeTARTS candy into my mouth and told me to bite down if I dared.

I dared. An immense explosion of chemical flavors raised not only the roof of my mouth but the very roof of my skull as well. I had tasted SweeTARTS before and thought I knew what to expect, but this was a new experience, more intense, more shocking and pleasurable. It started a shiver between my shoulder blades that spread up to the back of my head and ended in a whole-body shimmy.

"Are you ready for a brownie?"

"You baked brownies?" I asked, having already forgotten. My mouth was soon coated with a divinely comforting chocolate slurry, and my whole body felt young and at home.

The next morning, I felt entirely normal again, but I was not the same. I didn't know it then, but the entire course of the career I planned in psychiatry had shifted toward a fascination with addiction medicine.

How Changes in Brain Function Caused My Cannabis Experiences

Let's analyze my set and setting, and then trace the path of the cannabis from smoke in my lungs to a shower of THC in different areas of my brain that produced the high I experienced.

My attitude toward trying cannabis was largely positive, although I had to acknowledge some anxiety about the unknown. But curiosity and excitement easily outweighed any nervousness, especially with Tom in my corner. I was in a celebratory mood because I had recently received my undergraduate degree and I was headed toward medical school. My increasing distrust for the government as the Vietnam War escalated had justified a rebellious streak in my otherwise conventional personality. My mindset clearly led to positive expectations for the experience I was about to have with cannabis.

The setting was perfect. Tom provided strong social support for my decision. He was enthusiastic about his own experience with cannabis and reassured me that I had nothing to fear. He would not smoke with me in order to remain clearheaded. He asked about my expectations before guiding me into the experience, and he avoided describing how being high would feel in order to "let me have my own experience." Baudelaire would have approved of the physical surroundings – a fire glowing in the fireplace, ice water to soothe a throat not used to smoking, and even a "little music" pumped through his powerful stereo speakers.

The cough and rasping throat from sucking in hot smoke from burning vegetation is similar to standing too close to a campfire or smoking your first cigarette. The active ingredients in cannabis and tobacco differ (THC and nicotine, respectively), but otherwise, their smoke contains nearly identical toxins, including formaldehyde, benzene, ammonia, and carbon monoxide. The concentration of particulate matter, including tar, in cannabis smoke is 29 percent higher than in tobacco, and the total amount of particles inhaled from a typical joint is three and a half times more than in a tobacco cigarette. No wonder my throat hurt.

The process of inhaling cannabis smoke also differs from smoking tobacco. I took a two-thirds larger puff, filled my lungs a third more, and held the smoke in four times longer than tobacco smokers do. As a result, five times as much carbon dioxide entered my blood. If I had become a regular cannabis smoker, I would have inflamed the lining of my large airways and possibly begun to suffer from a chronic cough and bronchitis. However, tobacco smokers light up far more frequently each day, and eventually suffer from emphysema, heart disease, and cancer, while these consequences have not yet been found in moderate cannabis smokers.

The ice water quelled my throat, and I became so entranced by the dancing spires of flame that I relaxed enough to quietly watch them as my mind spun fascinating daydreams about what I was seeing. I did not reflect on what was happening to me until Tom drew me back into conversation. This brief description provides a lot to unpack and analyze. To begin, the deep relaxation I felt came from the impact THC had on two distinct parts of my brain, each being the infrastructure for a specific function, namely movement and emotion. Picture these areas of the brain as roads over which traffic flows. The road is like the brain infrastructure, and the traffic is the mental function enabled by the infrastructure. During a period of construction to repave a lane, traffic slows down, leading some drivers to feel frustrated and others to look more closely at the surrounding landscape. Each driver's personality uniquely influences the experience. A temporary change in the infrastructure of certain areas in the brain alters their functioning, and thus the experience they contribute to consciousness. THC's stimulation of greater-than-normal negative feedback in these two areas altered the chemical balance in them, and was thus mind-altering as well.

Our motor system has three interlocking layers: the planning, initiation, and fine-tuning of physical movement. Planning physical movement begins with developing an "image of achievement" in a group of neurons beneath the brain's surface called the basal ganglia. An image of achievement might be catching a ball or picking up your toothbrush. This image of achievement then activates the neurons in the cortex on the surface of the brain that control individual muscles. Electrical stimulation of different parts of this motor area causes contraction of the muscles each area controls, initiating organized, purposeful movement. The portion of our motor system located on the brain's outer layer is only moderately populated by CB1 receptors, but CB1 receptors are densely concentrated in the basal ganglia. Finally, the cerebellum, located at the back of the brain, fine-tunes our movements, calculating how fast to run and when to raise an arm to catch a fly ball, for example. The cerebellum's structure is well designed to provide fine motor control; a microscopic view of its neurons reveals an orderly array more reminiscent of a computer microchip than any other part of the brain. This structure calculates both where and when fine muscle movements should occur to bring an image of achievement to fruition. The cerebellum has an especially high concentration of CB1 receptors.

THC's strong and lasting activation of CB1 receptors in the motor system affects movement in two ways. The first effect occurs in the basal ganglia. Activating the large number of CB1 receptors here reduces spontaneous movement. The more THC is given to an animal, the more motionless it becomes. Gentle pushing does not rouse the animal; only vigorous or painful stimulation will get it moving. It is not paralyzed; it merely lacks any effective images of achievement arising from the basal ganglia. I was that inert animal as I lay comfortably motionless on the floor, wondering how I would ever be able to move again as a simple act of will. While I did possess an image of achieving a sitting position, THC seemed to limit this image's activation of my motor cortex. Couch lock, or being too stoned to get off the couch, occurs when the receptors in the basal ganglia are activated beyond their normal level. I found the extreme physical relaxation enjoyable and a welcome change from the fidgeting I often feel when trying to meditate or fall asleep.

THC's effect on movement arising from the cerebellum is seen in decreased fine motor control and an altered sense of time. Impaired fine motor control is demonstrated when THC slows a test subject's attempt to insert grooved pegs that need to be oriented correctly to fit into holes. My cerebellum's overestimation of time was consistent with multiple laboratory experiments that asked subjects to estimate intervals of time. The cerebellum is an important part of our brain's mechanism for experiencing clock time; too much negative feedback in the ECS within the cerebellum causes our experience of time to slow.

The deep, emotional relaxation I experienced came directly from THC's activation of CB1 receptors in my amygdala. This area of the brain, comprising an almond-sized collection of neurons located 2 inches above the corner of the eyes in the temporal lobes on both sides of the brain, is central to much of the cannabis experience. Electrical stimulation of the amygdala can evoke a multitude of different emotions, including rage, anxiety, a feeling of peace and calm, or a sense of divine presence and awe. The amygdala is also responsible for the fight or flight reflex. Experiences with cannabis vary; depending on the user's set, setting, and unique brain chemistry, THC's effect on the amygdala can cause either panic or relaxation. Luckily, I happened to have the right setting, temperament, and amygdala to respond to THC with deep relaxation and awe. I was later amused to find writings by Carl Sagan, the notable astronomer who co-wrote and narrated the award-winning 1980 TV series *Cosmos*. Under the pseudonym Mr. X, Sagan described his experience with cannabis in great detail and with deep scientific curiosity at a time before the keys to understanding cannabis had been discovered. He also found staring into fires when high to be "an extraordinarily moving and beautiful experience." The reason for his and my fascination with flames when under the influence of cannabis lay in the altered chemistry in the amygdala.

One important function of the amygdala is to compare what we are experiencing in the moment with our previous experience. When our current experience matches what came before, we notice it less vividly. When something new occurs, the amygdala adds a noticeable "zing" to the experience to alert us and draw our attention to its novelty. For example, if a tone is repeated at the same pitch and then suddenly changes pitch, our ears perk up. Our brains will begin to ignore the common tone, but when it changes, our amygdala will alert us by adding its zing to our experience of the tone. The way in which the tone changes is inconsequential; it is the change itself that matters. The amygdala acts as a constant comparator, waiting to call our attention to anything novel. Even the cessation of a constant stimulus, like a refrigerator's hum, can produce a zing to orient our attention to the change. Some people are drawn toward novelty, enjoy it, and seek out the experience. Others are more constrained in their reaction to novelty and draw back because they feel apprehension or anxiety. Intriguingly, this difference in temperament stems from genetically determined differences in the number of CB1 receptors in the amygdala.

The comparator function of the amygdala is influenced by cannabinoid chemistry. The bar for determining whether a stimulus is novel is regulated by the level of activity in the amygdala's ECS. When activation of the ECS is high, smaller changes trigger the alerting zing. Lower ECS activity means changes have to be greater to register as novel. THC's long and strong activation of CB1 receptors in the amygdala temporarily lowers our familiarity with common stimuli, which leads us to notice them anew. For example, imagine the small rainbow appearing on every bubble in soap suds. After childhood, most of us have become so thoroughly habituated to this rainbow that we no longer notice it. The delicate spectrum of color doesn't catch our eye as we routinely wash another sink full of dishes. When under the influence of cannabis, however, THC's action in the amygdala dishabituates us. The bar for experiencing the rainbow as novel is lowered and a zing is added, directing our attention toward it. We notice the rainbow with fresh eyes and are fascinated, re-experiencing the emotions we had as a child. We may even become childlike and playful with the bubbles. The entire event is delightful and captivating. This is how I came to see the dancing flames in Tom's fireplace as something new and deserving of close inspection. I was "stopping to smell the roses."

The rising of previously ignored experiences back into our awareness is often mistakenly identified as cannabis heightening our senses. However, objective testing of hearing and vision shows that we do not hear quieter sounds or see more dimly lit objects when under the influence of cannabis. Our sensory mechanisms are no more sensitive than usual. The difference in experience arises from the attention we give sensations when they feel new again, increasing the vividness of the stimuli. One lesson cannabis teaches many people is just how cloudy and dim their perception of their everyday world has become as a result of it becoming too familiar and routine.

My profound contemplation of the energy released by uniting oxygen and carbon as the flames danced in the fireplace resulted from my own idiosyncratic, scientific proclivity. Someone else would have had wildly different thoughts about the fire as a result of the same activation of receptors in their amygdala. Perhaps they would have ruminated on ancient cave dwellers' fascination with fire or their own guilt for releasing more carbon dioxide into the atmosphere. But regardless of anyone's particular musings, we would all be equally likely to struggle to remember the details of our experience, just as I quickly lost track of Tom's announcement that the brownies were ready. I had been so distracted by the SweeTART explosion in my mouth that I had entirely forgotten about the brownies. Carl Sagan wrote about experiencing similar memory glitches, acknowledging that most of the "amazing" ideas he had when high were either utter nonsense or quickly forgotten unless he wrote them down or shared them with someone else. Poor short-term memory is one of the most universally acknowledged effects of cannabis. It is common for people to lose their train of thought by the time they reach the end of a long sentence, which is often an occasion for gales of laughter.

The area of the brain responsible for short-term memory is shaped like a seahorse, which led early anatomists to call it the hippocampus – the Greek word for seahorse. Connections from the amygdala alert the hippocampus to a novel stimulus, and this activates the hippocampus to create a neural model of the stimulus. Once this neural representation has formed in short-term memory, it can then be uploaded into longer-term storage elsewhere. This is the basic mechanism of learning. Because the hippocampus is heavily endowed with CB1 receptors, our short-term memory is exquisitely affected by THC. The more active CB1 receptors are, the less effective the hippocampus becomes in forming short-term memory. The sensitivity of our hippocampus to CB1 activation plays an important role in the lasting effects of frequent cannabis use, explored in Chapter 13.

Baudelaire's "hope for a little music" is much easier to arrange with today's stereo systems. When my amygdala interpreted every note as novel, music became a vibrant, full-bodied experience. I don't know the strain of cannabis I consumed that evening, but it gave me both a mental and a body high. As I listened to Pink Floyd's highly electronic music, I could feel my nervous system responding throughout my entire body. I was connected to my physical being in a way I had never been before. My reveries about the sensation of sound occurring within my brain while physical pressure waves traveled through the air were a result of the idiosyncrasies of my own inclination toward scientific understanding. Experiencing the phenomenon of my mind projecting the sound out through the air still fascinates me in a way I imagine is similar to people who feel a phantom itch in an amputated leg. I rehearsed this insight enough at the time to remember it clearly to this day. Carl Sagan also remarked on how cannabis improved his appreciation of music by helping him hear the individual voices in a three-part harmony for the first time. Novelty.

The increased vividness of food is another example of how THC lowers the bar for novelty in the amygdala. The sharp, chemical taste of the SweeTARTS candy was more intense than I expected, and it felt as if I had never experienced the candy before. Sagan's delightful description of how the tastes and aromas of food emerge anew is an excellent example of dishabituation. Cannabis enabled him to experience what had become so common that it had fallen into the background, beneath conscious awareness. In his words, "I am able to give my full attention to the sensation. A potato will have a texture, a body, and taste like that of other potatoes, but much more so."

Tom's brownies illustrate something more than just the vivification of sensory experience. They also illustrate the impact of THC on appetite. It is well known that cannabis stimulates appetite, a phenomenon commonly called the "munchies." Many cannabis users describe not just the stimulation of their appetite but a craving for comfort foods. The source of hunger stimulated by cannabis can be found in a small collection of neurons deep within the brain called the hypothalamus, where hunger and satiety centers both exist.

CB1 receptors are more concentrated in the hunger center than in the satiety center. A French pharmaceutical company, Sanofi-Aventis, created a medication that caused weight loss in obese patients. The medication, called rimonabant, blocked CB1 receptors in the hunger center, thereby reducing endocannabinoid activity and decreasing hunger. When this benefit proved to last for a year *and* patients reported smoking less tobacco, it looked as though the company had struck gold. Unfortunately, rimonabant impacted more than just the hypothalamus. It also blocked receptors throughout the brain, resulting in serious side effects, such as severe depression in over 10 percent of patients. Rimonabant was withdrawn from the market, but its use did illustrate one very important fact: a well-balanced ECS is necessary for maintaining good mental and emotional health.

An Israeli scientist interested in appetite performed an illuminating experiment with the ECS. Ester Fride administered a dose of rimonabant to newborn rat pups in their first 24 hours of life. As a result, all the pups failed to suckle and died, despite their mother licking their mouths, which normally stimulates a newborn's sucking reflex. Rimonabant had inactivated the hunger center in their hypothalamus. A well-functioning ECS is necessary for the very existence of all mammalian species, as suckling soon after birth is essential. This association of endocannabinoid-evoked suckling and the comforting experience of a mother's milk suggests that THC may stimulate more than mere hunger. Perhaps it also arouses impulses toward comfort and bonding. Called the "Love Drug" during 1967's Summer of Love, cannabis has been seen as a prosocial drug in the USA ever since. In fact, a movement in the UK argues that supplying cannabis to inmates would reduce violence among prisoners.

There are still many unknowns about the relationship between cannabis and the brain. For example, why does using cannabis often result in laughter? There is no identified laughter center in the brain, so laughter is likely a complex social event involving surprise and pleasant incongruities. As such, laughter depends heavily on set and setting – a person's expectation and an appropriate environment for openly acknowledging and communicating absurdities.

Despite the remaining mysteries, a surprising number of the main characteristics of cannabis intoxication are explained by the impact of THC on CB1 receptors in the basal ganglia, cerebellum, amygdala, hippocampus, and hypothalamus. THC in the basal ganglia reduces spontaneous motor activity and quells physical restlessness. In the cerebellum, it impairs fine motor control and timing, leading to the overestimation of time intervals. In the amygdala, THC reduces anxiety in most people, while paradoxically raising it in others. Its impact in the amygdala also vivifies sensations by increasing their sense of novelty and stimulates a sense of awe and wonder. THC impairs hippocampal function, reducing short-term memory and learning. And in the hypothalamus, THC arouses the hunger center to seek primarily comfort foods.

Conclusion

The quest to uncover how THC works led to the discovery of our brain's own natural cannabinoid system. Before cannabinoid receptors had been discovered and Mechoulam found anandamide, we didn't know that this important neurotransmitter system existed. Once the ECS was discovered and examined, we began to understand its two primary functions: stability and flexibility.

Although stability and flexibility may initially appear to be opposites, they are important complements to each other. Stability comes from negative feedback by the ECS on other neurotransmitter systems, providing homeostatic control of the brain's chemical balance. The complex interplay of brain chemicals is like a sculptural mobile, designed to move freely in response to a breeze. The balance is delicate, and no element of the mobile can be permitted to dominate. The ECS maintains the activity of all other neurotransmitters within normal parameters, never too much and never too little. This delicate balance prevents any neurotransmitter system from dominating or becoming too inactive.

In an ever-changing world, flexibility is required to maintain stability. The willow's ability to bend in strong winds makes it more likely to survive a storm. Humans face many challenges that require the flexibility the ECS can provide. For example, increased cannabinoid tone in the motor system can help hunters avoid unwanted spontaneous movements while stalking prey. Flexibility in varying lengths of short-term memory is beneficial to accomplishing different tasks. Longer short-term memory is needed when trying to remember a phone number while you look for your phone. But performance in fast-moving situations, like a basketball game, may be improved by quickly forgetting what just happened and having the flexibility to respond to the immediate moment. Fluctuating levels of activity in the ECS adapt our brain to function best in response to changing demands. In the hypothalamus, the ECS modulates secretion of the stress hormone cortisol. The ECS thereby maintains our physiological stability by contributing to the flexible regulation of the body's stress response.

Raphael Mechoulam summed up what cannabis has taught us about the brain when he said that our ECS is involved in regulating nearly every physiological function in the body. This gives us even more reason to believe that our physical and mental wellness depends on a well-balanced, healthy ECS.

Sadly, I lost track of Tom after I moved west. He played an important role in my life by teaching me to respect the power of mind-altering drugs. All these years later, I still thank him for this perspective. Unfortunately, I learned a few years ago that he may not have remembered the lessons he taught me, as tobacco and alcohol shortened his life. May we all remember that eternal vigilance is the price of freedom.

5 PUTTING CANNABIS IN PERSPECTIVE

When Lynn went into her daughter Emily's messy bedroom to look for a magazine, she smelled the distinct odor of marijuana. After a quick look around, she found a sandwich bag of marijuana, a couple of joints, and rolling papers. She knew her daughter had tried marijuana before but thought it was only an occasional thing at parties. This stash looked a little more serious, and Lynn wondered if she should be worried. When asked about her use, Emily argued that everyone in her high school either smoked pot, vaped cannabis, or was lying. She insisted that her mom should be happy she'd never tried the hard stuff, like some kids were using. Lynn checked with the mothers of her daughter's two best friends and heard the same story. She decided to trust that Emily was telling the truth about kids her age. Both of Emily's friends were doing well academically and one was on the volleyball team, so Lynn felt there was no use in arguing.

When I asked Lynn if she had ever used cannabis, she said, "Sure, when I was young, but I grew out of it." Then I asked about her alcohol use. "Of course. Napa's got some of the best wines in the world." She and her husband maintained an extensive wine cellar and belonged to a wine-tasting club. She knew a lot about local wineries and had clearly studied the differences between their vineyards. She described her interest as a hobby. They usually shared a bottle of wine at dinner but added that they rarely got intoxicated. When asked if their friends were also into wine, she blithely said, "No, but they all drink something. No one has a problem with it."

People do not like statistics. All those numbers are dry, boring, and, for most of us, hard to understand or remember. Besides, we all know how statistics can be used to hide the truth and lie. Mark Twain popularized the clever saying, "There are three kinds of lies: lies, damned lies, and statistics." Then, when the science of epidemiology is introduced as the most reliable source for medical statistics, most people's eyes glaze over and they consider skipping the rest of the chapter.

Making Friends with the Science of Epidemiology

Let's start from a place of enough humility to admit how vast the world is compared with our own miniscule slice. There are nearly 330 million Americans, and nearly 8 billion people globally. The average person knows approximately 600 people in their lifetime. Most of these 600 are merely acquaintances, and only between 10 and 25 are known well enough to be deeply trusted. This means that each of us has direct experience with a very, very small sample of the whole population. If no one in your family uses cannabis, it is less likely that anyone in your small group of trusted friends will be a cannabis user. However, if a couple of people in your family enjoy cannabis or use it medicinally, it is more likely that others in your inner circle will also use cannabis. Our direct experience is an unreliable window into the wider world. While your direct observation may lead you to believe that very few people, or conversely nearly everyone, uses cannabis, this conclusion is highly biased by the narrow view we all necessarily have of the whole. Even asking a trusted friend for their observations won't get you very far out of your narrow box. The bottom line is that we cannot trust our own experiences to give us an objective view of the entire population.

This would be like taking a small handful of jelly beans from a 50-gallon barrel and concluding what the rest of the barrel contains. If you happened to grab a disproportionate number of green jelly beans because the barrel's contents had not been well mixed, you may end up with a wildly inaccurate idea of the color assortment of beans in the barrel. The simple truth is that we all lead statistically insignificant lives, and acknowledging this is a blow to our self-esteem.

So, how do we get beyond our limited experience in order to gain an accurate view of society as a whole? We rely on experts who have dedicated their careers to the laborious task of counting beans in the most objective ways science can devise. This sounds like we are being forced to accept experts' opinions on good faith, which is not often the best strategy for finding the truth, but it is exactly at this point that the scientific enterprise steps in to minimize the amount of blind faith demanded of us. If there were only one official bean counter and his or her results were declared to be the unarguable truth, science would not exist. That would be an *eminence*-based system and not an *evidence*-based one.

Fortunately, science involves a highly competitive community of researchers dedicated to improving the accuracy of counting beans. Each researcher's results and the methods used to obtain them are evaluated by other independent scientists before results are published for all to see. Then, other researchers strive to disprove or improve these published results in an unending process of challenging, confirming, and advancing each other's work. Science is conducted like an enormous game. Everyone agrees on the rules, and then they break their backs to one-up each other. At the end of the day, they often relax together over a good meal, while a few continue to argue bitterly about the others' mistakes. The banishing of opinion in favor of objective measurement is everyone's goal. Science is one of the most complex and noble enterprises the human species has created, even if its findings aren't always used for good.

With the scientific method in mind, let's use what researchers tell us about cannabis, its use, and its relationship to other drugs to gain a fair perspective on the society in which we live.

Measuring Cannabis Use

It's a complicated task to gather data about cannabis users because the US government considers all cannabis use to be illicit, which only means illegal. However, many states have enacted pro-cannabis legislation, deviating from federal policy. At the time of writing, there are 41 states with a population of 298 million people (93 percent of all US citizens) for whom medicinal cannabis use is legal by state law (although seven of those states permit only CBD), despite the fact that it remains illegal at the federal level. Furthermore, 18 states and the District of Columbia (with a combined population of 107.5 million adults, 43 percent of the US total) permit the legal use of marijuana for social/ recreational purposes, and more states are poised to follow suit. The country is clearly in the midst of liberalizing cannabis law, but there are no guarantees that we won't reverse course.

Despite discrepancies between state and federal cannabis laws, the federal government is still the best source for information about how many people use cannabis and how often. Every year, the US Substance Abuse and Mental Health Services Administration (SAMHSA) conducts an extensive survey called the National Survey of Drug Use and Health (NSDUH). In 2019, almost 70,000 Americans, aged 12 years old and up, were personally interviewed, reaching urban, suburban, and rural areas in every state. The 2019 NSDUH found that, among the 276 million

Table 5.1 *Percentage cannabis use by age groups*

Age (years)	Lifetime	Past year	Past month
12–13	3	2	1
14–15	14	12	6
16–17	31	25	15
18–20	43	33	21
21–25	57	37	24
26–29	60	33	22
30–34	58	25	16
35–39	56	21	14
40–44	51	16	10
44–49	47	14	10
50–54	52	12	8
55–59	54	13	9
60–64	57	14	10
65+	31	5	3

people over the age of 12 in the USA, 46 percent have used cannabis at some point in their lifetime. This means that 127 million people have violated federal law, which is reminiscent of the level of disregard for the law during alcohol prohibition. In the past year, 17.5 percent of respondents used cannabis, with 11.5 percent having used in just the past month. Among 12–17-year-olds, 16 percent have used cannabis at some point, 13 percent have used in the past year, and 7.4 percent in the past month. The use among people between 18 and 25 years old is 52 percent in their lifetime, with 35.5 percent during the past year and 23 percent during the past month. Clearly, not everyone uses cannabis, but a whole lot of people have, and still do. Table 5.1 breaks down use by age groups in greater detail.

One obvious fact jumps out when analyzing the data: most people begin cannabis use as adolescents or young adults. By age 17, half of one's peers who will ever try cannabis have already done so. At the same time, any adolescent who claims that "everyone uses weed" is simply not correct. The teens who have not experimented yet are actually the norm. When Emily tells her mother that "everyone smokes marijuana," she is more accurately describing her group of friends than the reality for all her peers. A second lesson from these numbers is that the frequency of use declines significantly after the age of 30, which is when family and career generally rise in priority. Finally, there is a steep drop-off in lifetime use for people aged 65 and older. People in this age group were born in 1956 and earlier, and it appears that the great cultural revolution in cannabis use brought about by the Summer of Love was limited in its impact and only enlisted greater numbers over time.

Cannabis is often labeled the most commonly used illicit drug in the USA. This claim is certainly true within the framework of federal law, which sees all cannabis use as illicit. Comparison with harder drugs also clearly shows the pre-eminence of cannabis. While 35.5 percent of 18–25-year-olds used cannabis in the past year and 23 percent in the past month, only 3.7 percent of that age group used opioids in the past year and 1.1 percent in the past month. Even fewer misused stimulants – 1.8 percent in the past year and 0.6 percent in the past month.

Another valuable survey, called Monitoring the Future, is funded by NIDA and performed independently by the University of Michigan Institute for Social Research. Each year, Monitoring the Future surveys the behaviors, values, mental health, and drug use of 8th-, 10th-, and 12th-grade students. In 2019, 42,500 students in 396 public and private schools across the nation were surveyed. Importantly, their results independently verified the

Table 5.2 *Results of the 2019 Monitoring the Future survey: percentage cannabis use in 8th-, 10th-, and 12th-grade students*

Grade	Lifetime	Past year	Past 30 days	Daily past 30 days	Ever daily for 30 days
8th	13.5	12	6.5	1.3	N/A
10th	31	29	18.5	4.8	N/A
12th	45	35.5	22.5	6.4	15

N/A, not available.

findings of the household survey conducted by SAMHSA, as outlined above (Table 5.2).

Initiation of cannabis use dramatically increases in frequency during the transition from middle to high school. By 10th grade, 80 percent of those who are going to use cannabis on a monthly basis during high school are already doing so. Daily cannabis use is also far more likely than daily alcohol use, which is reported in only 0.1 percent of 8th graders, 0.5 percent of 10th graders, and 1.2 percent of 12th graders. The advent of electronic vaping makes cannabis use far easier to conceal. In 2019, 9 percent of 8th graders, 22 percent of 10th graders, and 23.5 percent of 12th graders reported vaping cannabis, which means using high-concentration THC. Once again, the data confirm that only a minority of teens are using cannabis – not everyone. Even during the last year of high school, it is just as normal to have never used cannabis as it is to have used it.

These surveys are valuable because they settle arguments about average cannabis use. Mere opinions based on personal observations should not be seen as generalizable facts. Two things confirm the reliability of Monitoring the Future's data. First, several states conduct their own independent surveys and achieve similar results. California, for example, conducts the California Healthy Kids Survey (CHKS) yearly and,

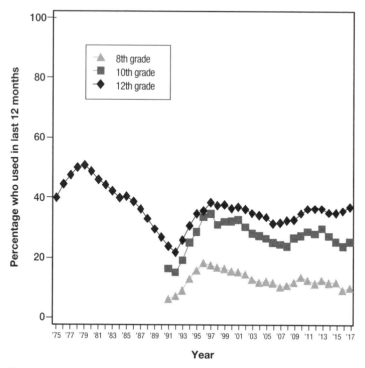

Figure 5.1 History of past-year cannabis use for 8th-, 10th-, and 12th-grade students.

although this survey observes 7th, 9th, and 11th graders, the CHKS data closely conform to Monitoring the Future's results.

Furthermore, the data reveal an extraordinary amount of consistency over time. The following three graphs are especially illuminating. The first graph (Figure 5.1) traces the trend in past-year cannabis use for 12th graders since 1975 and for 8th and 10th graders since 1991. Past-year use by 12th graders peaked in 1979 at 51 percent and then declined to 22 percent by 1992, largely due to increased law enforcement during the Reagan era and the "Just Say No" campaign. Use climbed steadily through the 1990s, leveling in 1997

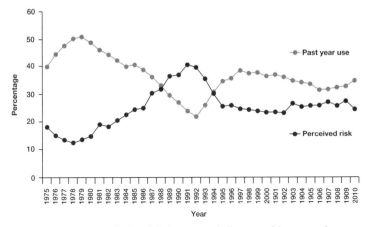

Figure 5.2 Inverse relationship between daily cannabis use and perceived risk in 12th-grade students.

and remaining relatively unchanged since, even as medical marijuana became legal in most states and several have legalized cannabis sales for social/recreational use.

The perception of risk associated with cannabis use by adolescents (Figure 5.2) generally has an inverse relationship to usage levels. As perceived risk climbs, usage drops, and vice versa. The peak level of use in 1979 was mirrored by the lowest level of perceived risk, while the lowest level of use in 1992 was mirrored by the highest level of perceived risk. However, persistent declines in perceived risk over the past decade and a half have not been as closely mirrored by persistent increases in use, perhaps due to a significant increase in the perceived risk of tobacco use, which very often accompanies cannabis use.

Figure 5.3 illustrates the trend in availability of cannabis, which is especially interesting with the passing of increasingly liberal cannabis laws. Since 1975, between 78 percent and 90 percent of 12th graders have said marijuana would be "fairly easy" or "very easy" to get if they wanted some. In

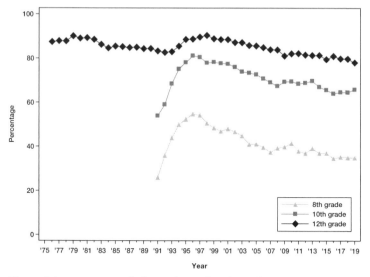

Figure 5.3 Percentage of 8th-, 10th-, and 12th-grade students who report marijuana is fairly or very easily available.

2019, that figure remained at 78 percent for 12th graders, stood at 66 percent for 10th graders, and fell to 35 percent for 8th graders. While it may seem shockingly high for 35 percent of 13- and 14-year-olds to report fairly or very easy access to cannabis, it should be remembered that older siblings are often the cannabis suppliers for those in early adolescence. The graph's trend line for availability is significant because it reveals no increase as states pass laws permitting medical and social/recreational use of cannabis.

Throughout my career in psychiatry and addiction medicine, I have almost never heard an adolescent complain about having to stop using cannabis because it was not available. Cannabis has been virtually universally available for any adolescent or adult motivated and clever enough to find it. This high level of availability, combined with many teens' desire to look cool and be accepted by their peers, likely convinced Emily that everyone her age used cannabis. Unless the government introduces extreme enforcement measures that most people would reject as seriously impinging on their civil liberties, cannabis will remain rated as "fairly easy" or "very easy" to find by teens. The responsibility for this availability rests solely on the shoulders of adults. If adults lost their current appetite for cannabis, there would be no cannabis industry. Teens do not grow, distribute, and sell more than a small fraction of what is available to them. The cannabis industry, both legal and illegal, is an adult enterprise, and as a result, adolescents have nearly universal access to cannabis. As I will discuss later, while adolescents have easy access to cannabis, access to treatment for those who are harmed is very limited.

Cannabis: One Among Many Substances People Use

Although cannabis is often described as the most widely used illicit drug, it is really only one leg on a three-legged stool. The other two legs are alcohol and tobacco. These three drugs constitute a triad because an adolescent's use of any one generally predicts use of the other two within a short period of time. The three run together so frequently that they form the initial context of many people's first use of cannabis. Figure 5.4 puts the three members of this triad into their proper perspective with the rest of the drug world.

The number of people 12 years and older who have used alcohol in the past month (48 percent of the population) abundantly laps the field and is nearly six times more common than cannabis use. It strikes me that people are generally comfortable talking about cannabis "use," but it may be jarring for many social drinkers to hear references

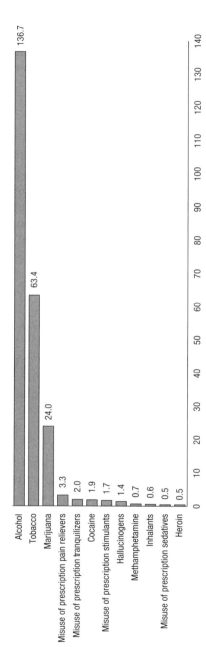

Figure 5.4 Past-month drug use in the USA. Estimated numbers of people refer to people aged 12 years or older in the civilian, non-institutionalized population in the USA. The numbers do not sum to the total population of the USA because the population for NSDUH does not include people aged 11 years or younger, people with no fixed household address (e.g. homeless or transient people not in shelters), active-duty military personnel, and residents of institutional group quarters, such as correctional facilities, nursing homes, mental institutions, and long-term care hospitals. The estimated numbers of current users of different illicit drugs are not mutually exclusive because people could have used more than one type of illicit drug in the past month.

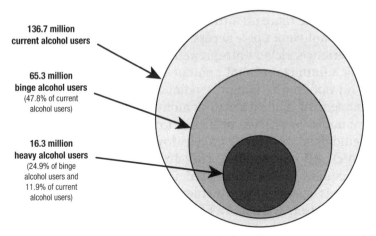

136.7 million
current alcohol users

65.3 million
binge alcohol users
(47.8% of current
alcohol users)

16.3 million
heavy alcohol users
(24.9% of binge
alcohol users and
11.9% of current
alcohol users)

Figure 5.5 Current, binge, and heavy alcohol use in persons age 12 and older.

to alcohol "use." People "have a drink" or a "few beers," but they do not often think of themselves as "using" alcohol. In contrast, it is quite common to hear someone say, "I could really use a drink" at the end of a long day. I contend that the only rational way to discuss alcohol is to simply see it as the most commonly used drug. Figure 5.5 shows that, of the 137 million Americans who used alcohol at least once in the past month, 65 million binge drank and 16 million qualify as heavy users. This means 47 percent of all those who drank alcohol in the past month binged at least once and 12 percent were heavy users.

Many object to lumping alcohol into the same category as drugs expressly used for their mind-altering properties or for getting high. Alcohol, it is often argued, is a beverage, a food. And so it is. Alcohol has calories like food, is enjoyed with meals, and can increase the appreciation of food. Except for lacking in calories, the same could be said for cannabis. But connoisseurs of fine wine, single malt whiskey, and craft beer argue that the motivation for their consumption is far more about taste than intoxication. While there is truth in this claim, there is also denial. If alcohol were not a necessary component of a drinker's experience, clever entrepreneurs would develop products that minimize alcohol content to make them healthier. I am not emphasizing the point that alcohol is a drug to condemn it but rather to demonstrate that cannabis and cannabis users have been irrationally and unnecessarily demonized. Attitudes taken toward one drug should match attitudes toward other drugs in the same category. Of course, cannabis is used in social and recreational settings specifically to achieve altered consciousness. If alcohol users were more honest, they would acknowledge that at least some degree of intoxication is desired, although they might euphemistically call it "relaxation," "stress relief," or "socializing." It's worth noting that binge and heavy alcohol users in the past month outnumbered cannabis users by roughly three and a half times, and people who use alcohol to that degree certainly intend to become intoxicated. The bottom line is that attitudes good for the alcohol goose should be good for the cannabis gander.

While the USA does not formally recognize a distinction between soft and hard drugs, many countries do, and cannabis is considered "soft." The Netherlands, for example, describes the distinction on its government website, stating that while soft drugs – such as hash, marijuana, sleeping pills, and sedatives like Valium – are not harmless substances, the risks are less serious than those associated with hard drugs, such as heroin, cocaine, amphetamine, LSD, and ecstasy. The Dutch classify drugs on the basis of level of health hazards, potential for addiction, and impact on public order. The boundary between soft and hard drugs is not distinct, so there is a lot of room for arguing whether any particular drug is soft or hard. Alcohol, for example, is clearly addictive, its association with violence is clear, withdrawal symptoms often require medical treatment, and an estimated 88,000 people in the USA die from alcohol-related causes annually, making it the third leading cause of preventable death. Nicotine, an even more addictive drug, is the leading cause of preventable death in the USA, killing 480,000 annually, including 41,000 deaths from second-hand smoke. Despite these facts, very few people would classify either alcohol or tobacco as a hard drug. Social and historical pressures contribute a great deal to society's assessment of the associated risks and subsequent classification of a drug.

In contrast, there are very few (if any) instances of people dying from an overdose of cannabis. While injuries and death from cannabis-related driving accidents have occurred, the number is difficult to determine with any accuracy and is undoubtedly far less than the number caused by drunk driving. Despite the relative safety of cannabis compared with the impacts of tobacco and alcohol, it remains categorized by the US Drug Enforcement Agency (DEA) as a Schedule I drug alongside heroin. In the eyes of the federal government, both cannabis and heroin are hard drugs posing equal health risks. To say that our drug classification system is irrational would be an understatement. Our system should reflect scientific facts but instead ignores research and is complicit with political forces. This state of affairs badly undermines confidence in drug education efforts.

The ultimate purpose of distinguishing between soft and hard drugs is to rationalize law enforcement and public health policy. Despite popular perception, all drugs are illegal in the Netherlands. The difference between soft and hard is that soft drugs are essentially decriminalized. The sale of carefully restricted quantities of soft drugs, while technically still illegal, is tolerated in licensed "coffee houses." This tolerance serves two purposes. First, it frees up law enforcement authorities to concentrate on the production, importation, distribution, sale, and possession of hard drugs, which are considered to be greater public health risks. Second, as the Dutch government recognizes the impossibility of eliminating all soft-drug use, tolerating the sale and possession of small quantities separates the soft- and hard-drug markets. People who choose to use soft drugs do not need to come into contact with the dealers of harder drugs. This separation protects the public while preserving enforcement resources to pursue the bigger and more important fish.

Although the US federal government makes no distinction between soft and hard drugs, a majority of states have decriminalized or fully legalized cannabis. Typically, decriminalization means no arrest, prison time, or criminal record for the first-time possession of small amounts of cannabis for personal use. In most decriminalized states, possession is treated like a minor traffic violation involving a ticket and a fine but, most importantly, no criminal record. Additionally, over 50 municipalities in a dozen states have enacted laws or resolutions decriminalizing minor cannabis possession offenses. The will of the people has turned against the War on Drugs.

Conclusion

There is a better way to respond to drug use than to wage war on drug users. While the USA is moving in the right direction by liberalizing cannabis laws, it does not lead the world in these efforts. The most extreme example of drug decriminalization exists in Portugal, which decriminalized the possession of small amounts of all drugs for personal use back in 2001. Those who violate the drug policy are referred to "dissuasion committees" comprising addiction experts and social workers who provide resources to help addicts move toward a healthier lifestyle. Police concentrate on suppressing illegal markets, not on punishing consumers. These policies have resulted in reduced harm from drug use compared with neighboring European countries. Portugal has demonstrated that a non-punitive, humane approach to drug use helps stabilize society – a lesson that puts both drug use and treatment in a new perspective.

Truly bold leadership would be necessary for the USA to take the same steps as Portugal. However, it is unlikely that even the boldest leadership will win the day until the public supports more humane treatment of drug users and demands a change.

6 CANNABIS CULTURE AND SPIRITUALITY

Jackson was bored with his massage therapy practice and was looking for something more interesting to do. Cannabis legalization had reawakened his interest in the use of natural, psychoactive substances as healing and spiritual agents. A once-a-month user of cannabis, he was enthusiastic about Johns Hopkins University's research on the potential mental health benefits of psilocybin, the psychedelic "magic mushroom." Jackson fondly remembered experiencing a spiritual awakening when he took LSD as a young man, but he had also seen the powerful drug send a friend into paranoid panic that lasted over a year. He believed cannabis offered a gentler experience and could be used therapeutically to open minds to a more spiritual life.

He grew increasingly excited about the idea of creating a spiritually focused counseling practice that incorporated cannabis-assisted healing. He began applying to clinical social work programs receptive to his plans, and he called me to ask for a letter supporting his idea. I was genuinely curious about his plans and asked what he thought cannabis could offer people seeking therapy.

My question released a torrent of enthusiasm. He said, "Most people's problems come from rigidly trying to force the same solutions that never work. They need to think more creatively and out of the box, and they need to stop trying to dominate their mind and nature instead of fitting into it. Cannabis can bounce people out of the narrow box their mind is locked in. It opens people to *experiencing themselves as an integral part of the world. We are all products of the natural world, and cannabis is God's gift to teach us how to live in harmony with nature, with each other, and with ourselves. It's the perfect medicine. Once people are open, therapy has a better chance of working."*

Motivations Underlying Cannabis Use

People use cannabis for many different reasons. My experience as a psychiatrist has taught me that all human behavior is overdetermined. This means that we rarely, if ever, do anything for only one pure reason. Almost everything we do simultaneously satisfies a large number of urges, ideals, logical reasons, practical concerns, and unique personality traits. Even paradoxical reasons can usually be found to be motivating some of our actions. Cannabis use is certainly determined by an abundance of motivations.

Motivations for non-medicinal cannabis users commonly include *enhancing* excitement and pleasant feelings, *coping* with stress and escaping personal problems (which is acknowledged as a motivation by one-third of cannabis users), increasing *sociability*, *expanding* self-knowledge, creativity, and spirituality, and achieving a different awareness of the world, often referred to as "expanding consciousness." All of these reasons for using cannabis combine with membership in a community committed to defending and promoting cannabis use to create what I call "Cannabis Culture." Unlike the scientific perspective, which strives for objectivity, Cannabis Culture focuses on the subjective experience and meaning of using cannabis. The vibrant Cannabis Culture community works to liberalize and normalize cannabis use and is organized around cannabis industry entrepreneurs who act as its leaders and spokespeople.

Public and Private Realms of Experience

It is easy to dismiss ideas about expansion of consciousness and spirituality from the materialistic perspective that guides hard science. I try instead to understand why cannabis is so often associated with spirituality and what people mean when they say that cannabis expands their consciousness. What is Cannabis Culture trying to communicate with these terms? Science has largely ignored, if not overtly discouraged, such subjective questions. However, a humanities course I took in college, called "The Public and Private Realm," taught that we all harbor a world of deep experience, an individual and private stream of feelings, urges, images, longings, and non-verbal, direct knowing. Our words and actions can never fully communicate our internal experience. It cannot be observed by others, and we are never given direct access to the inner, subjective lives of those around us. Our most intimate relationships come the closest to drawing another into our private realm, which gives them such precious importance to us. No matter how important this private realm is for molding our beliefs, actions, and sense of self, scientific methods of observation are largely impotent in the exploration of our subjective realities.

Spiritual/religious communities value this private realm of deep subjective experience more highly than material reality. From this perspective, importance is placed on our relationship with the infinite unknown and the mysteries still hidden beneath the surface of what is seen and objectively knowable. Spiritual practices remove humans from the weight of mastering the material world and right-size us into a more realistic perspective. Our infinitesimal smallness is felt at the same time as we feel woven out of the very fabric of the universe. Spiritual questioning pushes us to seek direct and deep experience of our connectedness to an inconceivably infinite whole.

Herein lies the promise of ultimate meaning, although few grasp more than mere glimpses of this truth. It is perhaps in our experience of deepening spiritual acceptance of our true place in the universe that we are most awestruck, and it is within this intense awe that our subjective experience is most like that of others. In other words, spiritual practice draws us into a communal, subjective experience of value and meaning. While science moves us toward an ever-deepening intellectual understanding of material realities, a vividly spiritual life can draw us into deeper levels of human experience. Both perspectives are important at different times and in different ways, and both are part of the human experience: the public and private realms. Just as both left and right feet are needed to walk effectively, attention must be paid to both objective and subjective experience if we are to make sense of the world's richness.

Becoming Aware of Constraints in the Private Realm

I described my first experience with cannabis in Chapter 4 for two reasons. I wanted to introduce several distinct aspects of being high in order to illustrate how THC-induced changes in function in different areas of the brain produce these unique experiences. I also wanted to illustrate the important experience of being unexpectedly knocked out of the box of my usual understanding of the world. Cannabis Culture sees this as being awakened from my straight way of thinking. Like the air we breathe, before my inaugural experience with cannabis, I assumed that the way I tasted food, the way I listened to music, and the way I saw myself in the world were the only ways. The air around us is so pervasive that we do not need to be aware of its presence to breathe. My "normal" experience was so consistently present that I had no idea it was only one possible way of relating to the world. Even though the altered consciousness of taste, sound, and self were drug induced, cannabis nevertheless revealed that awe had been missing and that other ways of experiencing the world were available to recapture it. People tend to be grateful for whatever revitalizes their childlike sense of wonder. The difficulty of maintaining access to our sense of awe was expressed in singer-songwriter Dan Fogelberg's lyric: "Mystery's a thing not easily captured, and once deceased not easily exhumed." This recapturing of possibilities is what Jackson believed to be an essential part of therapy and one that could be enhanced by cannabis.

My first experience with cannabis taught me I had been looking at the world through a narrow frame, a specific lens that determined my experiences. Up until that moment, I had been experiencing the tastes, sounds, and sense of self that I expected from past experience. This lens was dominated by the process of habituation and restricted my experience, robbing it of richness and limiting me to a rut defined by what I expected the world to be. Learning that an alternate frame of reference existed was like discovering for the first time that the air around me exists despite its invisibility.

Cannabis kicked me out of my box in a way alcohol never had, probably because alcohol is more of an anesthetic, a sedative, and soporific. It reduces the activity of all nerve cells, which initially lifts the user's mood by liberating them from anxiety and inhibitions, but eventually puts them to sleep. Alcohol puts us deeper into our box. Cannabis is different. I was fascinated by watching how introducing the plant's chemistry into my brain altered the workings of my mind without reducing consciousness. I was suddenly witness to the intimate connection between mind and brain, one of the greatest mysteries still eluding our understanding. I have my own unique way of expressing this fascination, and enough other people throughout history have shared their fascination that a culture has coalesced around cannabis for millennia.

Cannabis Culture Through Time

Advocates for the medicinal use of cannabis enjoy telling its long history of use in treating a wide variety of ailments, including diarrhea, pain, epilepsy, and inflammation. An equally long history of its use for transcending normal experience and seeking spiritual goals exists. The grave of a shaman buried in western China nearly 5,000 years ago contained over 1.5 lb (0.7 kg) of THC-positive cannabis among his relics. Over 3,000 years ago, the spiritual use of cannabis spread to the Indian subcontinent, appearing in Hindu scriptures describing its use by the god Shiva for meditation. Cannabis has been used ever since by ascetic holy men, in Hindu rituals, and as a drink concocted of ground cannabis flowers, milk, and spices sold in bhang shops, the oldest known continuously used cannabis product. Sacred texts from the ancient Zoroastrian religion in Persia describe its use, and Sufi mystics incorporated cannabis into their rituals. With their prohibition on alcohol, Muslims turned to hashish as their primary social/recreational drug. After Napoleon invaded Muslim countries with a group of scientists and anthropologists in tow, the use of cannabis as an intoxicant moved into Europe, and the French invasion of Algeria from 1830 to 1847 further increased the popular use of hashish. The Club des Haschischins' literary elite, artists, and scientists contributed to Cannabis Culture by exploring drug-induced experiences through eating amounts of hashish large enough to induce hallucinations. Of the experience, the philosopher Gautier said, "The bonds of matter and spirit were loosened." He said, "This is how souls must be in the world of essences. [...] I understood, then, the pleasure felt by spirits and angels moving in the ethereal regions." Throughout history, Cannabis Culture has comprised users seeking sociability, pleasure, medicinal benefit, and spiritual transcendence.

Cannabis Culture is far more diverse today. People motivated by politics, entrepreneurship, civil rights, opposing the drug war, criminal reform, and libertarianism have joined those advocating for its social/recreational use, medicinal use, and use as a spiritual aid. Cannabis Culture has evolved its own language, humor, etiquette, holiday (4/20), movies (e.g. Cheech and Chong, *The Big Lebowski*), art, music (best symbolized by the reggae genre), and literature (over 1,500 books on marijuana are offered on Amazon, in addition to novels that feature marijuana as an important part of the plot, such as *Invisible Man* and *Rule of the Bone*).

Marijuana brought into New Orleans from the Caribbean was adopted by Black musicians there as they were giving birth to American jazz. The new music spread to northern cities and into mainstream society, and most white Americans were oblivious to weed's influence on their entertainment. During the 1920s alcohol prohibition era, "tea pads" in Harlem apartments served as the cannabis equivalent of speakeasies. Radios and phonographs played the tunes that topped the Black hit list, including Louis Armstrong's "Muggles" (a popular slang term for marijuana well before J. K. Rowling's *Harry Potter*), Cab Calloway's "That Funny Reefer Man," Fats Waller's "Viper's Drag" (another slang term), and lesser-known artists' tunes such as "Smokin' Reefers," "Mary Jane," and the "Mary Jane Polka," all produced by major record studios. Even the white clarinetist Benny Goodman got into the act with "Texas Tea Party" and "Sweet Marihuana Brown." I still remember my mother gushing over Cab Calloway's energy and talent on the Ed Sullivan

Show back in the 1950s. Little did America understand that the flood tide of Cannabis Culture was soon going to be upon us.

The ripple of counterculture beatniks embracing cannabis during the 1950s was followed by the tsunami of the countercultural revolution of the 1960s, started by hippies and young anti-war protesters. Marijuana had breached the ramparts erected since Harry Anslinger's "Reefer Madness" campaign following the repeal of alcohol prohibition in late 1933. President Nixon saw marijuana as an existential threat to straight society. He conflated it with resistance to the unpopular war in Vietnam and politicized the issue to his own benefit. The buttoned-down atmosphere of the post-World War II years ended with a boom as Baby Boomers rejected the constraints of the 1950s. Modern Cannabis Culture was born.

Music was the powerful backbone at the core of Cannabis Culture as electrification of guitars energized rock and roll. In 1966, pot smokers eagerly misinterpreted Bob Dylan's lyric "Everybody must get stoned," and the Beatles' Paul McCartney wrote "Got to Get You into My Life" after being introduced to what he called the "mind-expanding" impact of marijuana, saying the song proclaimed, "I'm going to do this. This is not a bad idea." The love-rock musical *Hair* opened on Broadway in 1968, glorifying the younger generation's rebellion against conservative values. The legendary 1969 Woodstock music festival drew an enormous crowd of more than 400,000 people for 3 days of sex, drugs, and rock and roll; I fondly remember driving past the turn to Woodstock on my way to my brother's wedding, tempted to change plans, but ultimately continuing on, partly because we all had tickets to see *Hair* in a couple of days. It was a heady time for many in my generation who were coming of age and yearning for a deeper sense of personal freedom than our parents had known. Bob Marley's reggae music symbolized getting high for many pot smokers, and his image adorned posters and T-shirts as a way of identifying and unifying cannabis users. From "One Toke [inhalation] Over the Line" by Brewer and Shipley to "Roll Me Up and Smoke Me When I Die" by Willie Nelson (featuring Snoop Dogg, Kris Kristofferson, and Jamey Johnson) and beyond, music has consistently been at the core of Cannabis Culture.

Rastafarian Religion and Cannabis

No musician has epitomized the confluence of spirituality and cannabis more than the Jamaican reggae guru Bob Marley. The tightest connection of spirituality to Cannabis Culture in the Americas developed in Jamaica, where the Rastafarian religion emerged from a complex mixture of ethnic influences. Enslaved Africans brought to Jamaica by the Spanish were freed to fight the British invasion in 1655, and some escaped to the interior mountains, where they kept their African religion and mythology alive. The British then kidnapped African people from the Gold Coast to work their lowland sugar plantations and Christianized them over time. After the slave trade was outlawed in 1807 and Jamaican slaves were freed in 1834, an influx of indentured servants from India began arriving in 1845. Indian immigrants brought cannabis with them, and the use of ganja (the Indian term) spread throughout the island. Out of this complex ethnic, political, and herbal mix, a new, unique religion and Afrocentric social movement emerged in the 1930s: Rastafarianism. The term "Rastafari" derives from "Ras (i.e. prince) Tafari Makonnen," Haile Selassie's name before becoming emperor of Ethiopia. Selassie's pan-Africanism plays a major role in Rasta beliefs.

Often stereotypically identified with dreadlocks, reggae music, and fat blunts (hollowed-out cigars filled with cannabis), Rastas number over 1 million today and can be found around the globe. Rastafarian beliefs are based on unique interpretations of the Bible; believers worship a monotheistic deity that partially resides within each individual. Based on several Old Testament verses, such as Psalms 104:14, "He causeth the grass to grow for the cattle, and herb for the service of man," Rastas use cannabis as a sacrament to more directly contact the God within, thereby manifesting the divine gift of "peace and love." In addition to their theological beliefs, I learned of Rastafarians' focus on the African diaspora and enslavement at a beautiful display in Washington, DC's Smithsonian Institution. In "Redemption Song," Bob Marley sang, "Emancipate yourselves from mental slavery, none but ourselves can free our minds," beautifully encapsulating a dual meaning: that people of African descent are responsible for shedding the legacy of colonial oppression, and that cannabis connects people to their inner divine nature, which makes everyone worthy of freedom.

Cannabis and Spirituality

Cannabis Culture is a perspective, a lens through which the world is seen. The central belief in this perspective, particularly well illustrated by Rastafarianism, is that cannabis is an entheogen, defined in Wikipedia as "... a psychoactive substance that induces alterations in perception, mood, consciousness, cognition, or behavior for the purposes of engendering spiritual development." There can be no doubt that cannabis induces such alterations, nor is there doubt that many people attribute spiritual experiences to their use of cannabis. As spiritual experience exists in the private, subjective realm, it is impossible to argue on objective grounds that this belief is untrue. For the moment, it would be best to withhold judgment in order to understand why people believe cannabis is an entheogen, why they value it for this property, and how the physiological effects of cannabis chemistry contribute to these beliefs. After thoroughly exploring all facets of the topic, readers will be better prepared to discern whether the lens of Cannabis Culture's spiritual beliefs hold meaning for themselves.

A quick scan of the Internet provides countless anecdotes about why some people feel that cannabis aids their spiritual life. For example, Stephen Gray's book *Cannabis and Spirituality: An Explorer's Guide to an Ancient Plant Spirit Ally*, claims: "Truly a medicine for body and soul, one of cannabis's greatest gifts is its remarkable potential for spiritual healing and awakening." An anonymous quote from a survey on the spiritual use of cannabis sounds like the testimony of a born-again Christian: "Cannabis changed my life. It brought me into contact with something larger than life – a spiritual dimension to my existence. It made me realize what I now regard as fact: that there is much more to our human existence than we are usually aware of. This earthly life is only a small part of our true life, and to die from this world is only to return home." And in a quote that sounds reminiscent of Rastafarianism, the great country-western singer Willie Nelson stated, "I think people need to be educated to the fact that marijuana is not a drug. Marijuana is an herb and a flower. God put it here. If He put it here and He wants it to grow, what gives the government the right to say that God is wrong?" These sentiments are echoed in Jackson's belief in cannabis as a natural medicine.

While surveys find that approximately 25 percent of non-medicinal cannabis use is primarily motivated by spiritual exploration, many social/recreational users also note their appreciation for the spiritual aspect of their cannabis experience. Those who have primarily spiritual motivations for using cannabis commonly report experiencing "insight, connectedness, joy, love, and unity with transcendent forces." Carl Sagan typified this perspective when he wrote, "I do not consider myself a religious person in the usual sense, but there is a religious aspect to some highs. The heightened sensitivity in all areas gives me a feeling of communion with my surroundings." There is power in the word *communion*, defined as "the state of sharing or exchanging thoughts and feelings; the feeling of being part of something."

How Cannabis Stimulates Spirituality

There are two good explanations for this sense of communion, one psychological and the other chemical. At the psychological level, especially back in the 1960s when a new generation was coalescing its unique identity, there was the wonder of sharing the deeply subjective experience of being high. There seemed to be no need to explain what it felt like to be high to someone else who had experienced marijuana, and little way to explain it to someone who hadn't. The fundamental commonality of the experience, despite being so highly subjective, seems to breach the usual barrier to communicating such internal experiences. It was only much later, after talking to hundreds of patients, that I realized how different the experience and meaning of cannabis use can be from one individual to another. Despite these differences, Cannabis Culture is sustained by most initiates feeling an immediate common understanding and bond. Perhaps most obviously, there is often a shared understanding that much of what parents, experts, and the government have preached about the dangers of cannabis is simply not true. Of course, only time will tell whether some of the dangers will overtake some friends' lives, or even your own. Seeing through the dark veil thrown over cannabis and breaking out of an overly habituated straight experience (Bob Marley's mental slavery) creates a heightened sense of commonality and camaraderie among those who share the experience. In response to this commonality, I once wrote a naive science fiction story about a researcher who discovered that EEGs measuring the brain waves of people while high were all similar, as though being high were a state of global communion. This image illustrates how Cannabis Culture is a highly shared perspective that sees cannabis, cannabis users, and the world differently from straight culture.

On the chemical side is the question of whether cannabis is a "love drug" with the molecular capability to increase interpersonal connectedness. There is not a simple answer to this question. The hormone oxytocin is recognized as such a chemical, capable of increasing social interaction and bonding. Early research found different levels of oxytocin in two types of voles, a small rodent found in both prairie and mountain environments. Prairie voles have higher levels of oxytocin and are monogamous, mating for life. Mountain voles, in contrast, have lower levels of oxytocin and are promiscuous in their sexual activity. However, when mountain voles are given oxytocin, their mating behavior stabilizes and they behave like their prairie cousins.

In humans, the release of oxytocin is stimulated by social interactions, including hugging and breastfeeding; in turn, oxytocin stimulates social interactions. When rats are isolated, their oxytocin is reduced. When they rejoin their cagemates, oxytocin levels rise. (I am left wondering whether any scientists have been measuring human oxytocin levels during COVID-19 lockdowns.) It has been proven that oxytocin and the natural endocannabinoids are interconnected. When the rats were returned to their cagemates, anandamide levels in the reward center of their brains also rose, but this rise was prevented by blocking oxytocin's action. Socially induced increases in oxytocin drive the rise in anandamide in the reward center. However, increasing levels of anandamide in the reward center by interfering with the enzymatic breakdown of endocannabinoids produce prosocial behavior even if oxytocin is blocked. In other words, high levels of endocannabinoid activity in the reward center are essential to oxytocin's stimulation of social behavior. Increased oxytocin produced by a hug is only one link in a chain that releases the reward of social interaction. It seems likely that the combination of oxytocin and THC would provide powerful reward for personal interactions. For some users, the sense of communion is generalized beyond human interaction, as illustrated by Carl Sagan's description of an ineffable sense of communion with his surroundings. I personally felt such a communion once while lying on my back on a warm, sunny day, arms outstretched and fingers kneading through blades of grass. I suddenly imagined I heard the Earth purring as though I were lying on the head of a giant cat and scratching between its ears. I was enjoying the Earth and it was reciprocating. I experienced communion with the natural world, of which I felt myself to be one small part. While not a religious experience, it was quite spiritual, for I temporarily transcended my usual separation from the natural world. I suspect oxytocin was flowing and further augmenting the already boosted cannabinoid levels in my reward center.

While oxytocin and cannabinoids explain the boost cannabis gives to social connections, the plant has other important impacts on brain function that contribute to spiritual experiences. We can begin this story with the experiences of people with temporal lobe epilepsy. Scars in the temporal lobe can ignite electrical storms that evoke a range of out-of-body experiences, numinous space–time distortions, mystical and religious experiences, and a sense of intense meaningfulness and awe. Because the brain has no pain sensation, neurosurgeons have sunk electric probes deep into the brains of conscious patients to locate and remove the source of their seizures. As these probes stimulate portions of the temporal lobe, where the amygdala and its densely packed CB1 receptors are located, patients often report ecstatic experiences of a divine presence and profound feelings of transcendence. These experiences should not be interpreted as reducing spiritual and religious moments to mere physiology. Rather, we should conclude that our brain contains the machinery for creating consciousness of a variety of non-normal experiences. Whether it's the presence of God or a high dose of THC activating CB1 receptors that gives rise to a sense of divine presence, either experience necessarily involves our brain. Discerning the actual cause of a spiritual experience is difficult, although it is easier if you remember having recently smoked a joint. Many in the Cannabis Culture have developed spiritual practices and pursuits as a result of sensing a transcendence of self while high. This response enhances the belief that a mystical quality in the plant can change cannabis users in a positive direction. In *The Wisdom of Insecurity*, philosopher Alan Watts cautioned that while religion (or by extension, a drug like cannabis) can point toward a spiritual path, too many people suck the pointing finger rather than follow the path it points toward.

It is common for people under the influence of cannabis to be convinced of the certainty of insights gained while stoned. The impact of cannabis on brain function can provide a partial explanation for this certainty. Activity in an area called the cingulate gyrus generates awareness of making a mistake (see Chapter 13 for more detail). Overactivity in the error-recognition function of the cingulate gyrus leads to many of the maddening symptoms of obsessive-compulsive disorders. For example, an overactive cingulate gyrus can lead people to repeatedly check whether they have correctly turned off a light switch. Certainty eludes them as an inappropriate sense of error pervades their experience. CB1 receptors are concentrated in the cingulate gyrus. A dose of cannabinoids can reduce obsessing over having made an error, although tolerance soon develops if cannabis use is continued for this purpose. For the occasional user, however, intense activation of CB1 receptors in the cingulate gyrus may provide a gratifying sense of certainty to any insight. When high, no pesky sense of error lingers to contaminate the brilliance of an idea or the sense of its ultimate truth.

Spirituality involves transcending our ego in order to see ourselves in proper perspective to the universe as a whole. Time seems to stop when we are filled with the awe this inspires. The time distortion experienced by most cannabis users contributes to a sense that one is participating in a different realm of expanded experience. Most researchers believe the cerebellum is intimately involved in producing our sense of time, and unsurprisingly, the cerebellum is heavily endowed with cannabinoid receptors. When intensely activated, these receptors lead people to incorrectly perceive time intervals; what seems like 15 minutes may only be 5 minutes on the clock. Experiences that are not bound by the usual sense of clock time can feel more meaningful and have a more profound psychological impact. Because timelessness is a hallmark of spiritual experiences, time distortions with cannabis are often interpreted as lifting people out of normal time and transporting them to an altered reality.

A Cannabis-Assisted Spiritual Program

One does not have to attend services at a religious institution to realize that many people visit houses of worship for reasons other than spiritual enlightenment. They may hope that religious services will help them cope with stress, or they may attend out of conformity, because being part of a community enhances their life, or in search of prayer or healing for an illness. It may even be true that only a minority of congregants are seriously pursuing a primary goal of spiritual growth. Nearly everyone in attendance feels some spiritual boost, but the most intense experiences are likely felt by those with a more pervasive and intentional spiritual practice.

The same is true for cannabis users and spirituality. Although many users claim to receive spiritual benefit, only 25 percent are intent on fitting cannabis into their broader spiritual life. Surveys of individuals who use cannabis to improve self-awareness and achieve transcendence reveal a different attitude toward the frequency of cannabis use than is held by more casual social/recreational users. These users understand that too-frequent use leads to a less intense experience, and so use is paced to achieve the deepest impact. In a motivations survey, one social/recreational user explained, "I have had many spiritual experiences with cannabis, and continue to use it for this purpose, although my overuse has dulled the experiences a bit."

In contrast, those surveyed who have primary spiritual motivations for cannabis use say the following: "My personal experience with cannabis has been very helpful. When I don't use it for a week or two, I'm getting very good trips. It feels like during my trip a part of my brain gets unlocked." And, "Because it is very intense for me, I only do cannabis a few times every year. Also, it's my experience that if I do it too often it gets less intense, and therefore less meaningful for me. I want it to be a special, transformative, revelatory experience, and in order to give it the space it needs, I must portion it out."

I was never sure whether Jackson was primarily interested in spiritual counseling or psychotherapy. While there is an obvious crossover between the two and I frequently discuss spiritual issues with patients, therapists have a deep responsibility to know their patients well enough to ensure they would not be encouraging cannabis use in someone likely to substitute its temporary relief for the hard work of psychological exploration and change. The university studies of psilocybin that excited Jackson used a non-addictive drug normally unavailable to the public, so there is little worry of overuse. Cannabis, in contrast, is addictive (see Chapter 11) and would be freely available to his clients in California. Some people seeking therapy may experience worsening symptoms with cannabis use and may not have the good judgment to use it safely. While cannabis has undoubtedly had spiritual benefit for many, Jackson will need extensive professional training to possess the skill required to identify clients for whom cannabis would be appropriate. Additionally, he will need to follow his clients closely to be sure they use it safely, and he must contend with the influx of people primarily interested in getting high who will learn of his practice and seek him out for this purpose, as well as to justify their use.

Conclusion

I have paid a great deal of attention to the spiritual aspect of Cannabis Culture, both because this phenomenon intrigues me personally and because it permeates so many other elements of the culture. I am intrigued because the issue of cannabis and spirituality so graphically and immediately demonstrates the mysterious connection between mind and body. The intimate connection between the two is laid bare by cannabis. And yet, despite our scientific understanding of the physical mechanisms of cannabis's interaction with the brain, comprehending how brain activity, normal or altered, gives rise to consciousness and our subjective experiences remains a mystery. Directly and palpably experiencing this mystery is one of the pleasures known to those who have used cannabis.

Cannabis Culture's view of medicine exemplifies how a spiritual lens suffuses the culture's perspective. I have frequently heard cannabis advocates claim that *all* use of cannabis is medicinal. This has been said in earnest by many cannabis advocates, including those who run non-profit clinics for aged and impoverished patients, by combat veterans suffering from post-traumatic stress disorder (PTSD), and by medicinal cannabis dispensary retailers. This perspective is similar to the Native American concept of medicine, which begins with the basic principle that humans are an integral part of nature. Health is seen as a matter of balance between humans and nature, as well as between the natural and spiritual worlds. Within this perspective, medicine possesses the presence and power to restore balance in a person, place, or object. The word for medicine in Native American languages often also means spirit, power, energy, or mystic force. Cannabis Culture views the plant as an integral part of nature, imbued with the power to awaken spirituality in all those who consume it. The plant is capable not only of treating many ailments but also of enhancing wellness and balance between humans and nature and between our physical and spiritual worlds. Whether you agree with this core belief or not, it is important to understand how deeply it permeates Cannabis Culture and how passionately it is held.

The intensity of many cannabis users' belief in their right to consume the plant and its derivatives was demonstrated during cannabis prohibition by their willingness to defy legal authorities and risk severe punishment. Belief in this right currently aligns with a libertarian political ideology, and most libertarians support cannabis legalization whether they personally use or not. The cannabis industry, which is rapidly becoming Big Marijuana similar to Big Tobacco, is particularly forceful in its libertarian approach to free enterprise. Their goal is to normalize and increase cannabis use both for ideological reasons shared by other cannabis advocates and for thinly veiled monetary reasons. Mixed into this libertarian, free-enterprise philosophy is a strong push for promoting equity, which means taking pains to redress the racial injustice perpetrated by the War on Drugs. The goals of equity are to provide minorities access to the burgeoning cannabis industry's promise of wealth, and to expunge criminal records for offenses that no longer exist today.

Finally, Cannabis Culture defends the right for people to have fun the way they want to. For many, getting high is simply a source of pleasure with no essential difference from the role alcohol has always played. The majority of social/recreational use involves some form of entertainment. From getting high to enhance the opera, a rock concert, a trip to the ballpark, or skateboarding and video gaming, enjoyment is the goal. Just as Alcohol Culture includes everyone from beer swillers to elegant wine connoisseurs, Cannabis Culture includes everyone from stoners locked to their couch to those who describe the mysterious Canadian strain of cannabis called God Bud as "a potent, indica-dominant hybrid that provides a strong, euphoric high while tasting of tropical fruit with undertones of berry, lavender, and pine." Fun.

7 MEDICAL CANNABIS, PART I: CANNABINOIDS WITH STRONG SCIENTIFIC EVIDENCE

Stacey had been a brilliant professor of mathematics at UC Berkeley until her multiple sclerosis (MS) crippled her and drained her of energy. Unable to get out of bed without assistance, she studied the research literature about MS and decided to try cannabis to treat her painful and debilitating muscle spasms. When Stacey consulted me, I confirmed that cannabis had been proven to reduce muscle spasms for patients with MS, although its long-term use in elderly MS patients has also caused some intellectual decline. Only she could weigh the possible trade-offs. She decided to give cannabis a trial run and soon discovered that a couple of inhalations of marijuana purchased at a local dispensary allowed her to get out of bed shortly after waking up. The relief was life changing, but she intensely disliked having to smoke it and hated feeling high.

I had no way of knowing the THC:CBD ratio of the marijuana available at her dispensary, so I suggested she ask a compounding pharmacy to prepare a prescription with balanced THC and CBD to see if this would reduce THC's mental disturbance. The pharmacy was not able to use cannabis, but instead compounded an oral medication out of Marinol (the brand name for synthetic THC) and CBD. This worked well but too slowly; Stacey sometimes needed over an hour before she could begin her day. I suggested Sativex, which is a faster-acting nasal spray with a 1:1, balanced THC:CBD ratio. Unfortunately, Sativex is produced in the UK, and although it is available across the border in Canada, it is illegal to import into the USA. We were never able to find a legal way to get Sativex for Stacey, and she was physically unable to travel to Canada to smuggle the medicine back home with her. She eventually had to settle for a strain of marijuana that her dispensary claimed was relatively high in CBD.

Interactions between cannabis and the brain that produce a high are only one part of the story, and many would say a less important part than the potential medical uses of cannabis and cannabinoid-based medications. This and the following two chapters look first at benefits with strong scientific proof, then at benefits with highly suggestive preliminary evidence, and finally at the medical benefits attributed specifically to cannabidiol (CBD).

Anecdotes and Data

A review of the difference between anecdotes and data will pave the way for evaluating the objective reality of cannabis's health benefit claims. As a physician, I feel an obligation to understand both the science and humanity of medical practice. When called upon to testify before legislative committees, I have often felt frustrated by watching anecdotes trump data. Data are facts gathered by powerful scientific methods that have been developed over centuries. Science operates under an agreed-upon set of rules designed to remove mere opinion and unconscious bias based on religious or ideological beliefs as much as humanly possible. Most data come from accurate measurements, repeated enough times and confirmed by enough other researchers to eliminate mistakes. Anecdotes are individual human stories and testimonials. Data speak to people's intellectual understanding, while anecdotes speak more to our emotions. Data are convincing, but anecdotes can be more motivating. For example, a parent may tell their child that the average tobacco smoker loses 10 years of life expectancy. The child reckons that this average means many cigarette smokers lose less than 10 years and assumes, in their youthful invulnerability, they will be among those who beat the odds. However, when a parent describes how they had to watch their child's loving grandmother slowly suffocate from emphysema while pulling an oxygen tank behind her wherever she went, a graphic image is created. When the parent tells of the shock at finding their mother crumbled in a lifeless heap in the bathroom one morning with the disconnected oxygen hose wrapped around her legs, this has the real power to affect a child. Anecdotes tell vivid stories, while data are designed to wring out fallible human perspectives in favor of reproducible, measurable fact.

Understanding the difference between anecdotes and data helps establish the legitimate role each plays in our medical decisions. For example, during the early stages of the COVID-19 pandemic, some people claimed that hydroxychloroquine could treat, or even prevent, the virus. Encouraging testimonials were given by people who were convinced the drug had minimized their symptoms or got them out of the hospital sooner. President Trump spoke of taking hydroxychloroquine for 10 days after a possible exposure to the virus without suffering any negative side effects. Because it was demonstrably true that the first testimonial reported only minor symptoms, the second had only a short hospital stay, and the president did not contract COVID-19 after that exposure, the stories seem to support hydroxychloroquine's beneficial effect. But these are merely anecdotes, stories. A problem exists when people's hopefulness or scientific illiteracy confuses correlation with causation. Correlation means President Trump's taking the drug and not getting sick both happened at the same time – again, a story, an anecdote. It is just as likely that the president also ate a hamburger during the 10 days after being exposed to the virus. That would be another correlation, although obviously more frivolous. It took painstaking research adhering to standard scientific methods to tease out whether taking hydroxychloroquine helped the president stay healthy or whether his continued health was only a coincidence and unconnected to the medication. This research required double-blind studies in which researchers gave either the active drug or an inactive placebo to similar patients with the same level of exposure and illness. Neither researchers nor patients knew which pills were the real drug. Statisticians used complicated formulas to calculate how many patients needed to be studied to ensure that random variations in probability did not confuse the results. Finally, when it was revealed which participants received a placebo and which received the real drug, we learned that hydroxy-chloroquine had absolutely no influence on who became infected with the virus, how sick they became, or who recovered. Unfortunately, researchers also learned that more people taking hydroxychloroquine had serious side effects from their treatment than those who took the placebo. This is objective data. No matter how many times the experiment has been repeated, the result is the same. Hydroxychloroquine has no value as a treatment for COVID-19, as much as many people hoped it would. Worse still, it can cause serious side effects. While anec-dotes about hydroxychloroquine raised hopes, the scientific data established the disappointing reality. Although some people continued to tout the value of hydroxychloroquine, scientists know that no number of anecdotes ever trump data.

Data do not disprove anecdotes. The story that President Trump took hydroxychloroquine after a possible exposure to COVID-19 and did not get infected is still true. It just has no objective bearing on the value of the drug. Like many people do, he confused correlation with causation. Two events that seemed on the surface to be connected were eventually proven to have been a coincidence. However, medical anecdotes can sometimes have real value. They dramatize diseases and draw attention to the suffering they cause. This attention can increase support for funding research to find cures. Anecdotes can also provide potential clues about new treatments that deserve rigorous investigation. There have been anecdotes throughout history about using cannabis to treat diarrhea, and data gathered by the scientific method have now proven these anecdotes to be true. Science has even explained the mechanism behind this antidiarrheal effect. Our gut contains CB2 receptors that slow intestinal motility and calm the intensity of cramping when activated by natural cannabinoids such as anandamide, 2-arachidonoylglycerol (2-AG), or THC.

We should not blithely dismiss anecdotes. Folk medicine can guide research toward valuable discoveries, but over-eagerness to take anecdotes as factual truth can bias our medical decisions toward mere hope rather than hard fact, and this places us at risk of pursuing ineffective treatments. Clever marketing and snake-oil salesmen with more interest in financial gain than the well-being of patients often use testimonials and anecdotes to raise hope and manipulate the public. It is often impossible to distinguish between the naive enthusiasm of medical cannabis patients and pure entrepreneurial greed. As with virtually every new medicine, overpromising occurs and can become rampant through the sharing of anecdotes. I will restrict myself to following the data in this chapter.

History of the Medical Use of Cannabis

Before pharmaceutical companies made and advertised medications, folklore accumulated and passed on knowledge about the medicinal benefit of plants, including cannabis. References to the medical use of cannabis are found as early as 2900 BCE in China, and are as widespread there as in India, Egypt, Greece, and throughout the Islamic world. William O'Shaughnessy is credited with introducing the Western world to the medical benefits of cannabis. Born in Limerick, Ireland, in 1809, O'Shaughnessy received his medical education at the University of Edinburgh. Also a chemist and engineer, he entered service with the East India Company in 1833 and later became a professor at the medical college in Calcutta. While in India, O'Shaughnessy learned about the medical uses of cannabis and began writing papers documenting his scientific and clinical research on the plant. He validated folklore regarding its medical uses, discovered new benefits, and began recommending its use back home. His reputation was solidified when his cannabis studies revealed a host of new medical benefits, including relieving the pain of rheumatism, providing anti-epileptic value in infants, and treating the excruciating spasms of tetanus and rabies, although cannabis did not cure these illnesses. This remarkable man was eventually knighted by Queen Victoria for his contributions to the telegraph system in India.

O'Shaughnessy's promotion of medical cannabis in Europe occurred at the same time as the emergence of the Club des Haschischins in Paris. In an era with few remedies for pain and inflammation, cannabis tinctures and elixirs quickly became America and Europe's superstar patent medicines. In the early 1900s, when progressive political efforts to protect public health and worker safety combined with anti-immigrant and racial prejudice, the first laws were passed to regulate cannabis in the USA. California's pharmacy board led the way in 1913 by prohibiting the non-prescription possession of "extracts, tinctures, or other narcotic preparations of hemp, or loco-weed." The law was expanded 2 years later to include forbidding the sale of flowering tops and leaves. Over 2,000 legal cannabis extracts, tinctures, powders, and elixirs remained available for medical purposes, including over-the-counter, 1-ounce bottles of powdered cannabis extract from Parke, Davis & Company. The 1937 Marijuana Tax Act prohibited the sale of all cannabis, despite testimony from the American Medical Association (AMA) that they knew "of no evidence that marijuana is a dangerous drug." The AMA warned that prohibition "loses sight of the fact that future investigation may show that there are substantial medical uses for Cannabis." All patent medicines containing cannabis were subsequently removed from the US pharmacopoeia in 1942. Medical cannabis did not reappear in the USA until Cannabis Culture persuaded California voters to pass the Compassionate Use Act in 1996, some 54 years later.

With the relegalization of medical cannabis, it was finally time for a rigorous scientific evaluation of its medical value. Unfortunately, scientific studies have often been hampered by the federal Food and Drug Administration's (FDA) outdated and thoroughly unscientific classification of cannabis as a Schedule I drug alongside heroin and LSD, a category of drugs with high potential for abuse and no legitimate medical use. Placing cannabis on FDA's Schedule I continues to be motivated more by politics and anecdotes than by data.

Current Data Supporting the Medical Use of Cannabis

The most respected review of medicinal cannabis supported by strong scientific evidence is a lengthy report issued in 2017 by the National Academies of Sciences, Engineering, and Medicine entitled *The Health Effects of Cannabis and Cannabinoids: The Current State of Evidence and Recommendations for Research*. The title contains a subtle but important message: by reporting on both cannabis and cannabinoids, the National Academies are broadening the topic well beyond what is usually referred to as "medical marijuana." The true target of their interest is less cannabis itself and more the ECS and compounds that interact with the ECS throughout the body to produce medical benefits. Cannabis plant products are only one way to modify the ECS. As sucking hot smoke from burning flowers and leaves into your lungs is unlikely to be the best way to take medicine, safer and more effective means were bound to be developed. Extracting measured doses of active ingredients and creating new combinations is already replacing smokable marijuana. The future will bring a host of chemical modifications to the basic molecules found in the cannabis plant to increase efficacy and reduce side effects. Even medications that block ECS activity will be developed to reduce the symptoms of some diseases. For example, as raising cannabinoid tone with THC reduces memory, perhaps using CB1 blockers to lower cannabinoid tone might be found to help dementia and reverse memory loss. The cornucopia of cannabinoid-based medications waiting for us in the future is vast and exciting. As more are developed, the raw cannabis plant will eventually be relegated to the same anachronistic category as willow bark for pain relief, the original source of aspirin, and foxglove tea for heart failure, the original source of digitalis. The National Academies' report should be viewed as a snapshot in time. It identifies diseases for which there is currently strong scientific evidence of benefit from cannabinoids. It is far from the final word on the subject. We are still early in the modern history of cannabinoid therapeutics, and new research is being added every day.

A commission of scientists interested in medical cannabis and appointed by the National Academies reviewed over 10,000 journal articles to assess the quality of scientific evidence supporting the medical benefits of cannabis.

For example, double-blind, randomized studies are considered the gold standard and are given the most credibility, while open-label studies in which both researchers and participants know the medication being studied do not control bias as well and are therefore considered less reliable. If an open-label study is not randomized or does not use a placebo as a control, its credibility is even a notch lower. The commission evaluated the level of evidence in the reviewed articles and then compiled the results. The goal was to replace *eminence*-based medicine, meaning medical practice dictated primarily by prominent authorities, in favor of truly *evidence*-based medicine.

Conclusive or substantial evidence exists that cannabis or cannabinoids are effective for the treatment of:
1. Chronic pain in adults.
2. Chemotherapy-induced nausea and vomiting.
3. Spasticity produced by multiple sclerosis.
There is moderate evidence that cannabis or cannabinoids are effective for improving:
4. Short-term sleep problems caused by obstructive sleep apnea, fibromyalgia, and multiple sclerosis.
This list of health benefits documented by the National Academies is not very long and certainly would be seen as wildly incomplete by many medical cannabis advocates and cannabis dispensaries. The list is nonetheless highly significant for three reasons. First, conclusive evidence of benefit for chronic pain sufferers, particularly when the dangers of opiate medications have finally been recognized, is important enough by itself to be exciting. Second, the National Academies' report shines a bright light on the FDA's failure to follow the science, which punches another hole in the public's trust in their judgment and motives. Third, the report establishes the legitimacy of medical cannabis research. This research is important both to document additional illnesses that can be treated with cannabinoids and to discredit marketers' health claims

based on misleading anecdotes. We can only hope that the National Academies' recommendation for further research will not continue to go unheeded by those who ignore and deny science due to moral judgments, political expediency, or sheer ignorance.

The list also illustrates the harm already being perpetrated by the FDA's failure to remove cannabis from its Schedule I restrictions. Stacey lies in bed longer than necessary every morning, waiting for her marijuana with unknown levels of THC and CBD to unlock her legs from their spasms so she can begin her day. The science proves she is using a legitimate medication that provides significant relief, yet she is prevented from getting the standardized dose in a preparation that acts faster and spares her lungs that Sativex offers. While this superior medication sits on pharmacy shelves just across our northern border, Stacey is forced to use second best. She is victimized by a system that is still controlled by a legacy of past ideologies instead of objective science.

My optimism about the potential for treating a wide range of illnesses by modifying endocannabinoid activity comes from the large body of what is called preclinical research – basic laboratory, bench, and animal research – which necessarily precedes human studies. On the basis of basic research results, Raphael Mechoulam predicted that a treasure trove of medical benefits awaits discovery. The rest of this chapter reviews the basis for medical cannabis's proven benefits, while Chapter 8 presents Mechoulam's predictions for the future.

Pain

The Centers for Disease Control and Prevention (CDC) estimates that 50 million American adults (20 percent) suffer from chronic pain, with almost 20 million having high-impact chronic pain, defined as substantially restricting activities for 6 months or more. It is no wonder that a ready market existed for the promise of relief offered by pharmaceutical companies pushing opiates and over-the-counter non-steroidal anti-inflammatory drugs (NSAIDs, such as ibuprofen). The CDC recently reported nearly 47,000 opiate overdose deaths in 1 year. Safer treatment of chronic pain is clearly a crying need.

Chronic pain is by far the most common reason for the medical use of cannabis. On average, 90 percent of people using medical cannabis cite chronic pain relief as their primary goal. Critics suggest that, as pain is a subjective sensation for which there are no objective signs to observe or measure, it is the easiest excuse for accessing legal cannabis. In addition, the average medical cannabis user seeking pain relief does not resemble the average medical pain clinic population, being considerably younger and more likely to be male. While there are undoubtedly people who game the system merely to gain legal access to cannabis for recreational use, this is not the whole story. Medicare prescriptions for opiates are significantly lower in states with legal medical cannabis, and one medical cannabis dispensary's patient survey showed a 64 percent reduction in opiate use. In the face of America's ongoing opiate epidemic, access to cannabis for pain relief has proven to be a useful harm-reduction strategy.

Long used as a folk remedy for treating pain, the National Academies confirmed strong evidence that cannabinoids relieve *chronic* pain, as distinguished from the *acute* pain typical of sudden trauma or recent surgery. This distinction between acute and chronic pain relief stems from the existence of two distinct, overlapping, anti-pain mechanisms in our nervous system. Opiate receptors and their natural transmitters, the endorphins, are present throughout the nervous system and are most effective at dulling the acute pain of traumatic tissue injury, such as cuts, burns, broken bones, and surgery. Cannabinoid receptors and their transmitters, anandamide and 2-AG, also exist throughout the nervous system and are most effective at quelling chronic inflammatory and neuropathic (arising from damage to nerves themselves) pain.

Interactions between the opiate and cannabinoid antipain systems have also been shown in the treatment of unremitting pain from end-stage cancer. While morphine alone does provide significant pain relief, the side effects of mental dulling and serious constipation often limit the dose that can be tolerated. Combining cannabinoid medication with a lower dose of morphine can provide sufficient pain relief with fewer negative side effects. Mysteries still exist regarding the ability of cannabinoids to combat pain. For example, when both men and women are asked to report the first sensation of pain while holding their hand in nearly freezing water, only men experience a longer wait time before feeling pain after receiving a standard dose of a cannabinoid. It is unclear why men have an increase in their pain threshold under the influence of cannabis, but women do not. This is only one of many examples of gender-based differences in reaction to cannabis.

Everyone has a basic sense of what inflammation is: that red, swollen, hot, and often painful reaction to a sprained ankle or infected cut. The mechanism of inflammation and the role of our ECS in combating it is intriguing. The immune system is designed to protect and heal the body in response to injury or infection. Unfortunately, our immune system can do harm when overactivated, as occurs in some people with COVID-19. An overactive immune response to the influenza virus during the 1918 epidemic contributed substantially to excessive deaths among healthy young adults. The immune system can even misguidedly attack a body suffering from autoimmune diseases such as rheumatoid arthritis, causing painful inflammation and joint destruction. The levels of CB2 receptors and 2-AG rise in inflamed areas to regulate the immune system response. Adding cannabinoid stimulation to activate the increased population of CB2 receptors enhances their anti-inflammatory action. Similarly, drugs that interfere with the breakdown of 2-AG prolong its effect and provide another way to increase CB2 receptor stimulation to reduce inflammation. Billions of people around the globe already use this strategy for inflammatory pain relief without knowing it. NSAIDs, such as acetaminophen (also known as paracetamol and Tylenol) and ibuprofen, interfere with inflammation enzymes that destroy 2-AG, thereby increasing its anti-inflammatory effect. Every day, more than 30 million Americans take an NSAID to enhance their natural ECS's ability to soothe pain and inflammation stemming from injuries, headaches, arthritis, and other daily discomforts.

It is impossible for me to recommend specific cannabis products for pain relief, or for any other medical condition. Different cannabis dispensaries offer different products with different ingredients. While the budistas at your local cannabis dispensary may give advice on which of their products are best for a given ailment, none are truly qualified to diagnose medical conditions or to know for certain whether the wares they sell are the safest and most effective treatment for your symptoms. Also, the concentrations of THC and CBD on product labels may not be accurate. As many as 70 percent of products tested by an independent laboratory in California contained inaccurate labeling. The term "medical" when applied to cannabis should be interpreted to mean only that the product is intended for medicinal benefit, not that ingredients and dosage are standardized to the degree expected from medications dispensed by pharmacies. As a result, you and your doctor cannot be certain what is really in the "Purple Haze" or "Northern Lights" you can find at the dispensary. The cannabis industry still needs to mature a good deal before it reaches the level of consistency and reliability attained by the rest of the pharmaceutical industry.

Chemotherapy-Induced Nausea and Vomiting

The mustard gas used in World War I was vile stuff. After exposure, soldiers suffered blistered skin, blindness, scorched throats, lung damage, and vomiting. When tasked with finding an antidote in anticipation of combat in World War II, scientists discovered that the toxic gas attacks the fastest growing cells in the body. As cancer cells were known to grow wildly out of control, a version of mustard gas was developed to fight cancer, giving birth to modern chemotherapy. Unfortunately, medical research has still not found a way to eliminate the nausea and vomiting that chemotherapy causes. This miserable side effect is much more than an "upset stomach." Cancer chemotherapy can also cause prolonged retching, dizziness, light-headedness, trouble swallowing, skin temperature changes, nerve damage, brain fog, and a fast heart rate. Even the newest anti-nausea medications only relieve nausea and vomiting 70–80 percent of the time, leaving a lot of room for improvement. Anecdotally, cannabis has often proved useful when pharmaceutical drugs have failed to work, especially in patients not naive to its use. Some hospitals have quietly started offering private areas for patients to smoke their marijuana before receiving chemotherapy treatments.

Research has now shown that both THC and CBD play distinct roles in treating nausea and vomiting. THC's activation of CB1 receptors directly reduces nausea and vomiting. The cannabinoid blocker rimonabant eliminates THC's effect, which proves that regulating the ECS is central to THC's benefit. Experimental drugs that block the breakdown of anandamide also reduce nausea and vomiting, which further proves that the ECS regulates this physiological function. CBD, in contrast, does not significantly activate CB1 receptors. It reduces nausea and vomiting by activating a portion of the serotonin system, which is also central to the function of vomiting. The effectiveness of cannabis equals that of modern pharmaceutical drugs, but its side effects (getting high) are bothersome to some, so people with previous cannabis experience are better candidates for its use during chemotherapy. An added benefit for those who tolerate cannabis treatment is the ability to regulate its dose throughout the period of nausea and vomiting, along with the reduced anxiety cannabis can produce (discussed in Chapter 8).

A seemingly paradoxical symptom involving bouts of repeated, severe vomiting is sometimes seen in daily, long-term cannabis users. Weeks or even months of early-morning nausea and belly pain may occur before bouts of vomiting begin. It is likely that this condition, called cannabis hyperemesis syndrome, results from severe dysregulation of the ECS caused by changes in brain chemistry and physiology that accumulate during addiction to cannabis. It may be more a symptom of partial withdrawal than the direct effect of THC. In either case, hyperemesis again demonstrates that our ECS plays a robust role in the regulation of nausea and vomiting, exemplifying the biphasic nature of some of the effects of cannabis.

A biphasic effect exists when a high dose produces the opposite effect of a low dose, prominently seen in the calming effect most people feel from low-dose cannabis and the anxiety or paranoia seen with higher doses.

Multiple Sclerosis

MS is a degenerative brain disease of uncertain cause. MS is characterized by unpredictably waxing and waning neurological symptoms, including numbness, muscle weakness, and loss of or double vision. Spasticity caused by MS makes

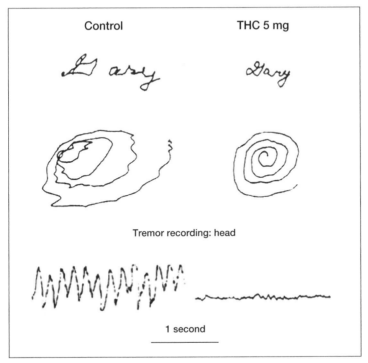

Control   THC 5 mg

Tremor recording: head

1 second

Figure 7.1 Multiple sclerosis patient before and after 5 mg of THC.

muscles feel stiff, heavy, and difficult to move. A typical spasm causes the sudden stiffening of a muscle, which can make an arm or leg jerk, leading to serious incoordination. Spasticity can be so severe that some MS patients like Stacey need medication just to get out of bed in the morning.

As described in Chapter 4, THC interacts with the brain's motor system to reduce spontaneous motor activity. Figure 7.1 graphically illustrates the dramatic impact that THC has on some MS patients' symptoms. On the left side is a patient's signature and drawing of a spiral and a straight line before being given THC. The right side, produced after

THC, shows remarkable improvement. It is not difficult to see how this improvement would contribute greatly to quality of life. Patients have told me they can take just a few puffs of marijuana as needed throughout the day to stabilize their spasms without feeling high.

Of course, all medicines have side effects, and cannabis is no exception. It is a very useful medicine for MS patients, but it comes with a particularly worrisome side effect. Unfortunately, cannabis use increases the severity of cognitive problems in MS patients. The disease leaves scars (plaques) throughout the nervous system and robs neuronal axons of their fatty insulation. This interferes with communication between different parts of the brain, and gradually leads to cognitive deficits. Cannabis use reduces brain volume faster than is normally seen in MS patients, and this correlates with increasing intellectual deficits. Cognitive side effects leave MS patients with a cruel dilemma. They have to choose between a higher quality of life now and the prospect of earlier cognitive difficulties later in life. There is no right answer. Each individual must act in line with what they most value. Physicians do have a right choice to make here, and that is to give every patient the objective information needed for them to make the best decision for themselves. Cannabis could be the ideal treatment for the disabling spasticity of MS for patients who can tolerate its potential side effects.

Sleep

Difficulty falling or staying asleep happens to 68 percent of Americans at least once a week, and 27 percent experience difficulties most nights. That the National Academies found even moderate sleep improvement with cannabis sounds like a godsend, but the situation is cloudier than we might wish. Their endorsement was carefully worded to avoid saying that cannabis treats sleep disorders. Instead, they said that there is only good evidence that cannabis offers *short-term* help with sleep disturbance associated with a few specific conditions: obstructive sleep apnea, fibromyalgia, and MS. Improved sleep is likely the result of the positive impact of cannabis on these underlying conditions. Because cannabis soothes chronic pain, reduces the inflammatory pain of fibromyalgia, and reduces muscle spasms in MS, it helps people with these conditions sleep better. The benefit of cannabis for obstructive sleep apnea is more difficult to understand and may come from a variety of directions, including reduced anxiety and physical restlessness.

The impact of cannabis on sleep is more complex than the National Academies' review of the limited medical literature. Too many people report anecdotal benefit from cannabis to ignore its current widespread use for insomnia. Chapter 8 delves into the existing evidence that suggests a legitimate role for the ability of cannabis to induce sleep, while also explaining some of the complexities that make it difficult to reach final conclusions about its value in treating insomnia.

Conclusion

The proof is in hand. Cannabinoids provide symptomatic relief of suffering from several diseases. Keeping cannabis on the FDA's Schedule I can only be supported by science deniers.

The same cautions need to be taken with cannabis as with any pharmaceutical drug. Only your physician is fully qualified to diagnose the underlying cause of your symptoms, and without an accurate diagnosis, purely symptomatic relief can permit serious illnesses to progress without proper treatment. Once your symptoms are diagnosed, your physician may not be fully informed about the safe and effective cannabis-based treatments that are available, given the long history of cannabis prohibition in the USA. As every medicine, including cannabis, has side effects, be sure to tell your doctor if you are using medical cannabis. It is the ethical duty for anyone who recommends cannabis for your symptoms, whether it is your physician or your local dispensary budista, to fully inform you about possible negative consequences. Unlike pharmaceutical drugs, there is no independent agency responsible for standardizing dose and guaranteeing the purity and identity of ingredients in cannabis products. All these concerns can be mitigated with improved physician training in cannabinoid therapies and stricter monitoring of cannabis products.

Until the regulation of medical cannabis catches up with the science, patients like Stacey will have to wait. The wait has already gone on too long for her.

8 MEDICAL CANNABIS, PART II: CANNABINOIDS WITH PRELIMINARY SCIENTIFIC EVIDENCE

Morgan had a classic case of attention deficit hyperactivity disorder (ADHD), although it had not been diagnosed until he was nearly 40 years old. A computerized test of his ability to withhold impulsive responses revealed that he performed no better than if he had been responding randomly. His ability to sustain concentration and avoid distraction was profoundly impaired. Morgan told me how this contributed to his poor work history. Despite doing well initially, he had lost several jobs when he got bored and began making careless mistakes. He felt he was intelligent and a hard worker, but things never seemed to work out – unless, he claimed, he used cannabis. He was convinced that smoking marijuana kept him calm and helped him concentrate, but he feared legal consequences if he had to continue relying on illegal dealers. He asked me to write a letter on his behalf, recommending he be given a state medical cannabis card.

I had never written a medical cannabis recommendation at that time, so I insisted he first experience a trial of at least two different medications considered the standard of care for ADHD. I wanted to be sure he was receiving the best possible treatment. Morgan reluctantly agreed and started using Adderall, which contains several different amphetamine salts. He reported no improvement with this first-line medication and complained that it increased his anxiety and physical restlessness. As he scored no better on the computerized assessment for ADHD, we went on to a second-line medication. Again, he reported no improvement and said he had recently received a negative evaluation at work. I insisted on one more trial – Marinol (pharmaceutical-grade THC) – in order to avoid the risks of smoking. He gave it a try but felt more anxious on this medication. Because his employment situation was becoming precarious, I agreed to write the medical cannabis recommendation if he agreed to see me on an ongoing basis so I could monitor the impact of restarting cannabis. Over the next few months, his employment situation stabilized, he reported feeling calmer, and eventually his computerized test improved modestly. I was never sure if his attentional difficulty improved because of the direct effect of cannabis on his underlying ADHD or because reducing his anxiety and physical restlessness made concentration easier, but in the end, it didn't matter. The quality of Morgan's life had improved.

Folk medicine is not a relic of a bygone era; it continues today. People use cannabis for a wider variety of health conditions than what the National Academies' report includes. Exclusion from the report does not mean evidence does not exist to support other conditions, only that research data are too preliminary and limited to draw reliable conclusions. Our understanding of cannabis is still evolving, so uncertainty must be tolerated as science fills in the gaps. Some early suggestive research will eventually verify the value of some treatments, while other research will be a dead end and offer no hard evidence for other anecdotal claims. The disease conditions explored in this chapter have early evidence of potential benefit from cannabinoid use. The suggestive evidence presented below is consistent with what is known about ECS function, but more research is needed to meet the accepted medical standards of proof. While many people have direct experience that makes them certain of cannabis's efficacy in treating the following conditions, the scientific community still needs more objective data to be convinced.

Science is more rigorously skeptical of bias than people who are suffering and desperate for relief. We need to pay attention to both perspectives. Folk medicine can point toward possible scientific breakthroughs, and science can prove, disprove, and improve folk medicine.

Two factors complicate the public's ability to evaluate health claims about cannabis. First, unverified and blatantly false claims about the ability of cannabis to cure everything from Ebola to Alzheimer's disease circulate on the Internet. University of Southern California researchers analyzed tens of thousands of tweets about cannabis and found that those sent by computer bots were more likely to contain claims of medical benefits without scientific evidence. This bot-driven social media traffic overwhelms accurate information on the Internet. Second, entrepreneurs have opened up a new avenue for promoting cannabis. In addition to recreational and medical use, new wellness promotions are appearing, especially regarding CBD. Wellness is defined as "being in good health," especially when this is actively pursued as a goal. Wellness activities include exercise, weight loss, and taking supplements, such as multivitamins, calcium, fish oil, and an expanding list of nutraceuticals. Supplements are not required to meet the FDA's standard of proof of safety and effectiveness as required for pharmaceutical medications, and they do not claim to treat any specific disease. They are promoted only as "supporting" mental or physical health – wellness. This laxity in legal regulation permits marketing of psychoactive THC and "non-psychoactive" CBD as a calming agent and sleep aid in some states. Promoting cannabis as a wellness product without scientific proof further confuses the public while profiting the cannabis industry.

Nevertheless, a good deal of exciting research exists regarding the potential for cannabinoid-based treatment of several important illnesses. Some of these uses are already popular, while others are not yet known or available to the public. This chapter reviews the available scientific information about the potential uses of cannabis to treat disease conditions not contained in the National Academies' report, and offers predictions for this age-old folk medicine's future uses.

Post-Traumatic Stress Disorder

The Mayo Clinic defines PTSD as a mental health condition triggered by either experiencing or witnessing a terrifying event. While it is natural to have temporary difficulties as the result of such an event, PTSD exists when flashbacks, nightmares, severe anxiety, and intrusive thoughts about the event persist for months or even years. As PTSD sufferers alternate between being overwhelmed and flooded with emotion or being numb and unfeeling, a variety of symptoms interfere with their lives, including depression, hyperarousal, memory and concentration impairment, sleep disturbances, digestive problems, headaches, and hypertension. Approximately 7–8 percent of adults in America will experience PTSD during their lifetime, and women suffer twice as often as men.

The prototypical PTSD sufferer in the public's view is the combat veteran, although this does not do justice to the rate and severity of PTSD suffered by victims of domestic violence and sexual abuse. A focus on veterans is particularly relevant to any discussion about medical cannabis as a treatment for PTSD because of the popularity of cannabis use among veterans and the number of studies analyzing cannabis use within the group. Because the federal government still prohibits cannabis for any use, Veterans Affairs hospitals are unable to recommend or provide cannabis, even in states that have legalized medical marijuana. As a result, several veteran organizations advocating medical cannabis use have sprung up, including

Weed for Warriors. Even as I write this paragraph, I have received an invitation to a cannabis information conference sponsored by the Veterans Cannabis Group. In order to understand why so many veterans with PTSD experience benefit from cannabis, and some of the limitations to this benefit, a few basic elements of the stress response must be understood.

When danger threatens, the amygdala sends signals to initiate our fight or flight response. A body in fight or flight mode directs maximum blood flow and energy to muscles and shuts down unnecessary functions, such as digestion. The amygdala accomplishes all this by activating the autonomic nervous system and initiating a cascade of stress hormones. Although the steps in this process are complex, the outcome is plain. The amygdala activates the hypothalamus to signal our sympathetic nervous system to increase heart rate and cause the adrenal glands to pump adrenalin into the bloodstream. This all occurs so fast that we can startle and develop clammy hands before even being conscious of the danger threatening us. If the threat persists, the hypothalamus recruits our pituitary gland to signal the adrenal glands to secrete the master stress hormone: cortisol. Cortisol raises blood sugar for maximum energy and prepares the body to heal any injuries. The whole stress response is normally self-limiting. A sudden fear that we have forgotten to mail our income tax return on time can activate the fight or flight response, with all its hormonal consequences. But once we remember it was mailed yesterday, the neural and hormonal stress response quickly fades. However, when our stress response is intense or continuous, as it is in combat situations, it overwhelms normal self-limiting influences. It is under these conditions that PTSD can develop. Once PTSD sets in, the full stress response continues to recur in reaction to even small reminders of the original trauma.

In a person suffering from PTSD, the amygdala remains hyperactive, ready to trigger fight or flight at a moment's notice, even when momentary circumstances only vaguely resemble the original trauma. Scientific research has clearly shown that a dose of THC quickly suppresses neural activity in the amygdala. As cannabis has an unmistakable benefit for most PTSD sufferers, it has become accepted wisdom that cannabis treats PTSD.

In addition, research also shows that the process of forgetting painful memories is controlled by our ECS. When rats are trained to seek shelter whenever a bell rings to signal an incoming electric shock to the floor of their cage, and then the shock stops following the bell, researchers measured how long it takes for rats to stop reacting to the bell. This research is an example of classical conditioning using a negative stimulus, followed by the extinguishing of the conditioned response. When given THC, the rats stop their fearful reaction to the bell sooner than those not given THC. When given a drug that blocks cannabinoid receptors (i.e. rimonabant), rats take much longer to stop fearing the bell. Our natural ECS is important for reducing our reaction to painful memories. Put another way, our ECS is critical for converting painful experiences into memories rather than allowing them to be re-experienced over and over. It should not be surprising that veterans are less bothered by intrusive, painful re-enactments of past trauma when they use cannabis. PTSD could be thought of as a failure of the ECS to quell the fear felt when remembering a traumatic situation.

The Trauma and Stress Support Centres run by the Canadian Armed Forces Mental Health Services gave a synthetic cannabinoid similar to THC (nabilone) to veterans with PTSD who were still having nightmares after conventional drug treatment. A remarkable 72 percent experienced less intense nightmares or a cessation of nightmares altogether with the cannabinoid treatment.

Unfortunately, the Centres did not control their study with a placebo, so the improvement could have been due to an infusion of hope brought by starting a new drug treatment. The power of a placebo to instill hope should never be underestimated. The Centres' study is a perfect example of potentially important data having less influence because of a low-quality research design. A similar study conducted 5 years later (2014) in New Mexico, also marred by the lack of a control group, found a 75 percent improvement in PTSD symptoms in veterans treated with medical marijuana. Just as no number of anecdotes rise to the level of data, it is also true that no amount of low-quality research rises to the level of higher-quality data.

As we know, all medications have potential side effects, and cannabis use for PTSD is no exception. Cannabis addiction, called cannabis use disorder (CUD), is a potential side effect with real-life consequences (see Chapter 11). According to the National Center for PTSD, more than 40,000 veterans were seen by the US Department of Veterans Affairs in 2014 with both PTSD and cannabis addiction. When people with cannabis addiction reduce or stop their cannabis use, amygdala activity rebounds above normal levels for a while, which increases PTSD symptoms. Fortunately, there are ways to quell ECS hyperactivity in the amygdala without using THC and therefore without risking a rebound increase in amygdala activity. For example, some drugs under development have been shown to reduce the breakdown of anandamide. Raising anandamide levels reduces activity in the amygdala without THC's side effects, including addiction. Even with an effective, non-psychoactive alternative available, not all PTSD sufferers would be willing to abandon cannabis. The seduction of the high from cannabis, with its general emotional numbing (see Chapter 13), is likely to make cannabis the drug of choice for many.

Gastrointestinal Disease

The oldest historical mentions of the medical use of cannabis involved gastrointestinal (GI) illnesses, particularly diarrhea. I was schooled in the effect of cannabis on the gut by one of my patients, a true child of the Summer of Love. Although she originally sought my counsel for difficulties in her relationship with her adult daughter, she soon told me of her unusual bowel habits, which included not having had a spontaneous bowel movement for several years. She relied on daily coffee enemas to remain comfortable. Her history of cannabis use was extensive – heavy, daily use for over 30 years. She had been under the care of an internist known for strongly advocating medical cannabis who had been encouraging her to increase her use as a natural balm for her worsening arthritis. While cannabis had taken care of her arthritic pain, it had wreaked havoc on her gut. Her colon had been rendered flaccid, lacking all muscle tone. Only the direct stimulation of caffeine in her enemas enabled her bowels to move.

A quick review of the literature revealed the mechanism of the antidiarrheal action of cannabis. Raphael Mechoulam began unraveling this story when he isolated the second natural cannabinoid neurotransmitter, 2-AG, from dog intestines. CB1 and CB2 receptors and anandamide were also soon found throughout the GI tract, from stomach to small and large intestines. Increasing cannabinoid tone with THC or elevating anandamide levels by giving a drug that blocks its breakdown can slow gut motility. Reducing cannabinoid tone by using rimonabant increases motility to such a degree that patients given the drug for weight reduction often complained of diarrhea. These basic cannabinoid dynamics in the gut suggest a variety of ways to treat GI diseases by modifying ECS activity. As many people object to THC's side effects of dizziness, dry mouth, fatigue, drowsiness, and altered mental state, its use to reduce overactive gut motility is limited. And rimonabant's side effect of depression limits its value in treating constipation. However, a cue could be taken from the treatment of opiate-induced constipation. The medication naloxegol (Movantik) combines an opiate blocker with a molecule that prevents its absorption from the gut into the bloodstream. Without absorption into the blood, the opiate blocker's uncomfortable psychoactive side effects (causing withdrawal in opiate users) are avoided. This same strategy could permit THC and rimonabant to be used to treat diarrhea and constipation, respectively.

Because the ECS is such an intimate part of the GI system, cannabinoid-based medications are a logical choice for potential new treatments for a variety of conditions, including chronic constipation, diarrhea, gastroesophageal reflux (GERD), irritable bowel syndrome (IBS), and inflammatory bowel disease (Crohn's disease). There was, however, only one effective treatment for my patient with a flaccid colon. The only cure for her profound constipation was total abstinence from cannabis. Rimonabant could have given quicker bowel relief but at the cost of intolerable withdrawal symptoms from cannabis (see Chapters 10 and 11). She agreed to extended residential treatment for her cannabis addiction, and her bowel function spontaneously returned to normal after 3 months of abstinence.

Bone Fractures and Osteoporosis

Mechoulam's interest in the medicinal uses of cannabinoids led him to investigate their role in bone health. Two of his colleagues discovered that THC, and especially CBD, reduced the healing time for standardized bone fractures by 30 percent. This benefit is achieved because bones contain two cell types with opposite functions, and both types contain cannabinoid receptors. One line of cells builds bone, while the other line of cells breaks bone down. Proper bone health requires a balance between the two cell types. Following a bone fracture, cells that build bone naturally increase their activity, and additional cannabinoid stimulation further activates their ability to build bone. Research is underway to investigate whether animal studies can be translated into new treatments for human trauma victims.

A seemingly random observation led Mechoulam to a deeper understanding of the role of cannabinoids in bone health. He noted that Greek women have 50 percent less osteoporosis than northern European women, and when he looked at dietary differences between the two groups, he found that the olive oil used more extensively in Mediterranean areas contains a molecule nearly identical to anandamide. This molecule, oleoyl, stimulates the activity of bone-building cells in the same way anandamide does. He then proved that oleoyl reverses bone-density loss in an animal model of osteoporosis. More than half of Americans over 50 (44 million people) have either lower-than-normal bone mass (osteopenia) or frank osteoporosis. The Medicare costs of treating osteoporosis and fractures was estimated at $22 billion a decade ago, and this provided treatment to only half of the elderly suffering with osteoporosis. Mounting evidence suggests that cannabinoid-based medications could make substantial contributions to bone health, especially in women, reducing the incidence of hip fractures that so commonly result from osteoporosis, while also reducing the time for healing all bone fractures by nearly a third.

Head Trauma, Stroke, and Heart Attack

Imagine yourself rushing to the hospital in an ambulance, your chest feeling painfully squeezed and short of breath.

Or perhaps you're feeling confused and paralyzed on one side of your body. You are gripped by fear as medics monitor your blood pressure, give oxygen, and start an intravenous drip. Then they inject the latest emergency medication into your vein: a cannabinoid-based wonder drug. Stoner fantasy or possible future reality?

Such a scenario is more likely than it sounds. Research in this area began with the observation in animal studies that the level of 2-AG in the brain rises tenfold within hours of a blow to the head. Administering a dose of 2-AG to rats soon after head trauma reduced brain swelling and damage. In fact, this single dose of 2-AG led to increased recovery 24 hours later and greater return of function after 3 weeks. Other studies have looked at similarly beneficial effects of cannabinoids when blood flow to the brain or heart is temporarily blocked, as occurs in strokes and heart attacks. In rats, a dose of CBD administered after 30 minutes of blocking blood flow to the brain, interrupting its critical supply of oxygen, showed reductions in swelling and brain damage. Cannabinoids also show benefits in rabbits after a 90-minute blockage of a coronary artery depriving a portion of the heart of oxygen. Will stroke and heart attack victims someday receive an emergency infusion of cannabinoid-based medication after being given a clot-busting drug to protect tissue from ischemic damage? This scenario seems more likely in light of the FDA's approval of a CBD-based solution used to bathe organs during transport to a transplantation center. CBD's ability to protect organs in transit from being damaged by insufficient oxygen is detailed in Chapter 9.

Neurodegenerative Disorders

A variety of degenerative diseases attack nerve cells in both the brain and spinal cord. These devastating illnesses still bedevil researchers, and little effective treatment has been discovered after years of research. Nearly 6 million Americans over the age of 65 (1 in 10) suffer from Alzheimer's disease. From the onset of difficulty remembering recent events, symptoms progress to include problems with language, disorientation, mood swings, behavioral problems, profound dementia, and loss of motivation, self-care, and bodily functions. The disease progresses over an average of 3–9 years. Nearly 1 million Americans suffer from Parkinson's disease, including heavyweight boxing champion Muhammad Ali and actor Michael J. Fox. Symptoms of Parkinson's begin in the motor system, including tremors at rest, muscle rigidity, and slower and decreasingly fluid movement, leading to difficulty walking. Advanced stages of the disease can include dementia and even hallucinations. Huntington's disease is a fatal, inherited disorder that affects 30,000 Americans, the most famous being the folk singer Woody Guthrie. As brain cells gradually die, subtle mood and cognitive symptoms progress, coordination is impaired, and jerky movements destroy physical abilities until a person is unable to even talk. Another 30,000 suffer from amyotrophic lateral sclerosis (ALS), also known as Lou Gehrig's disease after the famous New York Yankees baseball player who was diagnosed with it. As motor neurons in the spinal cord die, muscles weaken and atrophy, leading to difficulty walking, swallowing, talking, and breathing. Effective treatment for any one of these terrible diseases would relieve unimaginable suffering created in patients.

   Research on these neurodegenerative diseases is limited by the difficulty of finding equivalent animal conditions. However, because these illnesses are so dire, cannabinoids have undergone human trials but failed to produce any consistent benefits. However, these trials only focused on the ability of cannabinoids to control specific symptoms, and not whether worsening of the disease was slowed over time. More sophisticated ways of elevating ECS activity, such as blocking the breakdown of anandamide and 2-AG, have not yet been tested.

It seems like wishful thinking to hope that the direct effect of cannabinoids or activating the ECS could help these destructive diseases. And yet, despite failing to provide any symptomatic relief, there are reasons to believe cannabinoid-based medications could influence the basic mechanisms of cell damage caused by these diseases. Although each neurodegenerative disease has its own unique cause – including genetic mutations, metabolic problems, environmental pollutants, and possibly even viral infection – ultimately, they all produce the same basic chain of events that damages nerve cells: excess free radicals, inflammation, and toxic neuronal overexcitation.

The very phrase "free radicals" sounds dangerous, and they can be. The term refers to atoms and molecules with an electron energized to combine with nearby neighbors. Cells are damaged when free radicals combine with their DNA or a vital protein. Highly reactive free radicals are naturally produced as a byproduct of the metabolic process. The primary free radical in the body is oxygen. In the air, two oxygen atoms grab onto each other and occupy their available electrons. Just as a campfire produces heat by breaking oxygen pairs apart and combining each atom with carbon in the wood, our cells have the machinery to combine the oxygen in our blood with fuel contributed by what we eat. The release of energy is controlled by a complex series of small steps that allow the cells to harvest the energy being slowly released. When we are healthy, our bodies can quickly scavenge any solitary oxygen atoms that escape this controlled process. When oxygen radicals become free, they quickly combine with other molecules, thereby transforming them into free radicals with a charged electron in a damaging chain reaction.

The control of oxygen free radicals is particularly important for brain health. Although only 2 percent of the body's weight, our brain's energy needs are so great that it uses 20 percent of our inhaled oxygen. This leads to a high concentration of free radicals in the brain. The damage done by oxygen free radicals is called "oxidation" (similar to the oxidation of metal, or rust), and the tissue damage done is called "oxidative stress." Molecules capable of combining with and neutralizing free radicals are called "antioxidants." Anandamide and 2-AG are antioxidants that contribute to the scavenging of free radicals. THC and CBD are also powerful antioxidants. They grab onto oxygen free radicals and prevent them from doing damage. The antioxidant properties of cannabinoids contribute to their potential use as neuroprotective agents and suggest the possibility that cannabinoid-based medications might eventually slow the progression of neurodegenerative diseases. It is equally possible that more effective cannabinoid antioxidants will be developed with fewer side effects.

The anti-inflammatory property of cannabinoids was established earlier in relation to chronic pain and head trauma. While CB2 receptors are normally found primarily outside the brain, we know that their presence inside the brain quickly increases after head trauma. Their number likewise increases in neurodegenerative diseases. Increasing CB2 receptors in the brain promotes neuronal survival by combating inflammation.

A third neuroprotective property of the ECS is illustrated by its interactions with human immunodeficiency virus (HIV), the virus that causes AIDS. The most common type of HIV, HIV-1, produces toxins that damage neurons by overexciting them. The ECS regulates neural activity by generating negative feedback, quelling increased activity. Anandamide and 2-AG activation of CB1 receptors can therefore reduce toxic neuronal excitability and increase cell survival.

We now know that the ECS has a spectrum of neuropro-tective properties, including reducing oxidative injury, inflammation, and toxic levels of neuronal excitability. These properties offer extraordinary potential for developing new medications to treat the devastating effects of neurodegenerative disorders. Because these disorders cause neurons to suffer from a combination of damaging forces, a combination of protective effects is needed, a combination uniquely provided by the ECS. However, such treatments are only potential at this point. Even if they eventually prove useful, it is unlikely they will cure the underlying causes of these diseases.

Cancer

Few health claims for medicinal cannabis evoke as much excitement and interest as its potential to cure cancer. The thought of cancer is terrifying and has led to a variety of phony panaceas, from macrobiotic diets to extracts from fruit pits (the laetrile craze). Compassion for people suffering from cancer contributed to California's 1996 choice to relegalize medical marijuana for symptomatic relief of the pain and fear cancer brings, chemotherapy-induced nausea, and often-profound weight loss. Scientific evidence has proven these benefits to be genuine. Many Californians across the political spectrum supported the Compassionate Use Act after 54 years of medical cannabis prohibition, precisely because they saw it relieve suffering in a family member dying of cancer. Anecdotes of shrinking tumors and cancer cures have also circulated widely, but there has been no scientific verification of whether cannabis actually played a significant role. As powerful as personal tales of cannabis cures may be, testimonials are not as important as objective data with controls that avoid bias and coincidence. Unsubstantiated tales of miracle cures in a Tijuana cancer clinic that involve smoking marijuana or receiving blood transfusions from guinea pigs may be true, but how can we be certain? They may be born more out of understandable hope than out of reality.

At the same time, basic laboratory research does seem to offer glimmers of hope. Cannabinoids inhibit and sometimes kill a variety of cancer cells grown in Petri dishes and reduce the growth and spread of some cancer cells implanted in animals. For example, treatment for a very aggressive form of brain cancer (glioblastoma multiforme) is studied by giving experimental drugs to mice after tumor cells have been transplanted into them. Both THC alone and an equal mixture of THC and CBD inhibited the growth of these transplanted glioblastoma cells. This sounds encouraging and justifies further research, but is the slowing of progression because of a direct impact on the cancer cells, or is it due to a reduction of inflammation that weakened the defenses of cells surrounding the tumor? Research needs to explore every possible explanation before we can be certain of the role cannabinoids might eventually play in cancer treatment. CBD reduces the toxic effects of a common chemotherapy drug used for breast cancer, making the patient better able to tolerate the drug.

While there is a trickle of data from basic bench research suggesting that cannabinoids may inhibit some tumor cells and enhance some current first-line therapies, hard evidence for a potential role in cancer treatment is scant. For the time being, it is best to rely on cannabinoids only for symptomatic relief, and not to substitute cannabis for current, more effective treatments. It can be difficult to temper hope with realism, especially when cancer poses a mortal threat, but acknowledging our disappointment with the inadequate state of cancer treatment can prevent us from the indignity of being preyed upon by delusional or cruel entrepreneurs during the final stages of our life.

Ethics and Medical Cannabis

The era of unregulated patent medicine was first curbed during Teddy Roosevelt's progressive reform movement in the early twentieth century. The Pure Food and Drug Act of 1906 created government oversight to protect the purity and safety of products being sold to the public. Modern descendants of patent medicines are found on over-the-counter pharmacy shelves, in the nutraceutical supplement industry, and now again in the cannabis industry. A constant theme throughout the history of patent medicines is the direct marketing of healthcare products to customers whose right to purchase them is aggressively protected. This theme reflects the essence of free enterprise, the American way of business. Although pharmaceutical medications are also directly and prominently advertised to the American public, their availability is controlled by physicians who are licensed and whose professional conduct is monitored. Most notably, your doctor is prohibited from profiting from medications they prescribe, which prevents a massive conflict of interest that would open the profession to the corrupt practice of prescribing unneeded and expensive medications to line their own pockets. It is simply unethical for the prescriber of a medication to also profit from its sale.

Because cannabis remains illegal under federal law and the DEA license necessary for physicians to prescribe medication is federally issued, no doctor can prescribe cannabis. Only a limited number of cannabinoids have received FDA approval, including THC (Marinol, Dronabinol), CBD (Epidiolex), and nabilone (a synthetic cannabinoid). Sativex (1:1 THC:CBD) is available in the UK but awaits approval in the USA. The most a physician can do is recommend medical cannabis in states that have legalized its sale. In these states, a physician's letter of recommendation permits patients to grow, purchase, possess, and use cannabis. In states that already legalize adult use of cannabis, a letter of recommendation from your doctor has little legal bearing. In this case, it only memorializes that you have consulted with a physician regarding the wisdom of using cannabis for a medical purpose.

Standards of care exist for doctors recommending the use of medical cannabis, especially in states that limit cannabis use to specific diseases. If you consult with a doctor regarding medical cannabis, it is useful to know what to expect. The accepted standards of care include the following:

- A formal physician–patient relationship should be established.
- A relevant history and review of systems should be conducted.
- A good-faith physical examination should be conducted.
- A diagnosis should be established.
- A treatment plan should be developed and discussed.
- Informed consent should be obtained after discussion of risks and possible adverse side effects.
- Measures of treatment effectiveness should be agreed upon.
- Ongoing monitoring of your illness and response to treatment should occur.
- Medical records should be kept.

These standards of care increase the likelihood that a proper diagnosis of your illness is made and the full range of possible treatments is offered, as opposed to what occurs at temporary cannabis events where nurses in short, pink uniforms meet people seeking a medical recommendation, and a 15-minute, one-time meeting with a doctor is performed. These standards are important for assuring proper diagnosis of what ails you, avoiding delay when serious illness needs prompt attention, and not taking too much medical advice from someone in a dispensary who wants to sell you a product. Unfortunately, these standards are rarely enforced by state medical boards and do nothing to guarantee that your doctor is well educated about cannabis. For physicians to improve their scientific understanding of cannabis, they might turn to my previous book, *From Bud to Brain*, which provides healthcare professionals with the research information needed to provide unbiased, objective answers to your questions.

Finally, a serious breach of ethics has been built into the very structure of the medical cannabis dispensary system. After patients receive a letter of recommendation from their physician, they are free to purchase any strength of cannabis medication, in any formulation, for any purpose, and as often as desired. If similar dispensaries were established for Prozac, permitting any dose, frequency, and purpose a customer desired with approval from a physician seen no more than once a year, the entire enterprise would be considered unduly dangerous and a shill for pharmaceutical companies. The entire medical cannabis industry has been caught by current legislation betwixt and between. Cannabis is either a legitimate, powerful medication with significant potential adverse effects, or it isn't. Claims of important medical benefits, which have now been verified, are not consistent with the laissez-faire distribution system currently allowed. Once the federal government permits the prescription of medical cannabis, three advances will likely occur. First, more rigorous standardizing of ingredients and dosing will be established. Second, medical cannabis will move into existing pharmacies, thoroughly disrupting current medical cannabis dispensaries. And third, health insurance will begin covering medical cannabis. The consequences of full integration of cannabis into medical practice will completely transform the current status quo.

Conclusion

Raphael Mechoulam's conclusion that the ECS participates in nearly every physiological function in our body lends credence to the possibility that medications modifying ECS activity could affect the course of multiple diseases. Science has already borne this out for some diseases and will prove it for others in the near future. Until then, it is good to remember that truth in advertising is difficult for people eager to make a buck. Despite how exciting the possibilities for medical cannabis seem to be, maintaining healthy skepticism is only realistic. As far as I can tell, the cannabis industry has earned no more right to be trusted than the pharmaceutical industry has. As always, *caveat emptor* – buyer beware.

Doctors need to remember Morgan's dilemma. The benefits that cannabis provided for his ADHD fell outside the boundaries of current medical knowledge and practice, but careful investigation proved these benefits were real. My obligation was to ensure that he received the most effective treatment available and to provide access to this treatment if I could. Progress in medicine requires both rigorous adherence to scientific methods and the humility to acknowledge that there is always more to learn.

9 MEDICAL CANNABIS, PART III: CBD FACTS, FADS, AND POSSIBILITIES

Jevon had the most difficult sleep disorder I have ever treated. He had used Klonopin, an addictive benzodiazepine, for years with some success. Even with the drug, he tossed and turned for hours most nights before finally falling asleep for a few short hours. Some nights passed without a moment of sleep. He began increasing the dose when it stopped working in order to get a little rest, and when it stopped working altogether, he had to go through uncomfortable withdrawal before it worked again. When he sought my help, I slowly withdrew him from the Klonopin and advised him never to use it again. I sent him for an evaluation at a sleep disorder clinic but received no better understanding of his sleep disorder and only the standard suggestions for medications. We eventually eliminated the addictive Klonopin and developed a nightly cocktail of several sleep medications, each at a relatively low dose. On his new regimen, Jevon averaged 6 hours of uninterrupted sleep with only a rare sleepless night. He felt markedly improved, although still not fully normal.

Some time later, I received a phone call from Jevon asking if he could try adding CBD. Several friends told him CBD solved their occasional sleep difficulty without any side effects, and the Internet made CBD sound like a perfect solution. He was enthusiastic to try it if I thought it was OK. I gave him the go-ahead and asked him to text me every morning for several weeks so I could monitor the effect. Jevon reported great success in the early days, almost 8 hours of sleep a night, but then the effect became more variable. By the 2-week mark, the benefit had all but disappeared. I was never sure how much of the initial benefit was due to CBD and how much was a placebo effect due to his high level of enthusiasm for a new medication. We left CBD as an agent he could try from time to time to see if it had its initial effect again.

Several months ago, Jevon proudly called me to report a different success with CBD. He had adopted a small rescue dog. The poor thing had been badly abused and was left with an even higher level of anxiety than is characteristic of such small dogs. When reading about CBD on the Internet, Jevon had seen advertisements of CBD-infused treats for pets. A few articles mentioned using CBD for anxiety in dogs. He called his veterinarian to ask if this claim was legitimate. The vet told him that CBD works as well for dogs as Prozac does for humans, so Jevon gave it a try. His dog soon calmed enough to make a noticeable difference, and the effect has lasted.

CBD is simultaneously the least understood cannabinoid chemical and the most hyped product in the new cannabis marketplace. The Harvard Health Newsletter estimates 2021 CBD sales to be $2 billion, and *Forbes* magazine predicts that CBD product sales will reach $20 billion by 2024. In the midst of the CBD gold rush, factual information about this intriguing molecule is very difficult to sort from fancy. There are good reasons for the public's relative lack of understanding about what CBD is, how it works, and what effects it produces, all of which are quite different from THC. The science of CBD is far more complex than THC, and scientists' understanding of CBD is less complete. Still, what is known is exciting and important to grasp.

In the hierarchy of marketing persuasion, factual information is less convincing than anecdotes, and personal testimonials are the gold standard. As a consequence, the public has been barraged with emotional appeals about CBD. One user wrote, "[CBD] is the best thing ever! I have rheumatoid arthritis and have tried many medications.

On my 5th day after starting this I felt better than I have in years!!! THANK YOU!!" Another said, "Since starting … CBD oil, I feel so much better mentally and physically. I've gotten myself back and it's a great feeling! My anxiety has decreased significantly and I feel so much calmer!"

While it is undoubtedly true that these customers have experienced highly pleasing results, they offer no concrete information guaranteeing similar benefit. They offer hope, and marketing firms like Strategic Factory claim that such testimonials generate 62 percent more revenue.

Before further examining the faddish quality of today's CBD industry, let's first examine what is known about this important element of cannabis's chemical stew. What is the history of CBD, what established facts do we know about its action in the body, and what reasonable potential exists for its medical benefits?

A direct descendant of President John Adams, chemist Roger Adams began studying marijuana in 1939, 2 years after it had become illegal in the USA. A year later, he isolated CBD from Minnesota wild hemp, and eventually he learned how to modify CBD chemically to synthesize THC. Working with the defense department to create a "truth serum," he administered elements of marijuana to soldiers and scientists working on the top-secret atomic bomb project. The search for a truth serum failed, but he did learn enough about the plant's pleasurable qualities to earn Harry Anslinger's hostility. The technology did not yet exist to isolate THC from the plant itself or to analyze the molecular structure of CBD, keeping the discoveries Raphael Mechoulam achieved over two decades later just out of reach for Adams. Mechoulam determined the exact structure of CBD in 1963, a year before he isolated and analyzed the structure of THC.

Research on CBD initially took a back seat to THC because its psychoactive effect is much less intense. At most, CBD has a very mild anti-anxiety calming effect for some people. Later, however, CBD became more inter-esting when its ability to modify THC's impact was discov-ered. Early studies of THC were confusing because samples of marijuana with equal amounts of THC often gave differ-ent results. This variability was due to the different amounts of CBD present, not because of CBD's direct action, but rather because of its modification of THC's impact. THC alone is more activating, often producing more anxiety than when consumed in whole-plant prep-arations. Animals given THC are more sensitive to fear-based learning, and THC alone is more likely to produce paranoia. Adding CBD to THC creates a more balanced, mellow high with less anxiety and paranoia. CBD modifies THC's impact by attaching to CB1 receptors in a way that changes their shape. When THC binds to a receptor with this altered shape, its impact is both lessened and changed in complex ways.

When we ask how CBD alone affects the body, we are faced with its involvement in over 65 different molecular interactions without any way of knowing which are most important. Diving into this rich array of CBD actions very quickly rises to a level of science geekiness capable of over-whelming even the most interested reader. A few key examples illustrate the dizzying complexity still waiting to be sorted out by scientists. As CBD alters the shape of both CB1 and CB2 receptors, it also modifies the effect of anandamide and 2-AG. CBD also changes the shape of some serotonin receptors, which may account for its anti-anxiety effect. It increases the level of anandamide by interfering with the enzyme that breaks anandamide down, and it interacts with temporary receptors that appear in inflam-mation. The bottom line is that only one thing about CBD is clear: we do not yet know exactly how CBD works!

CBD comes from three sources, the first of which is the cannabis flower. As described in Chapter 2, both CBD and THC come from the same precursor in the flower, cannabigerol, or CBG. Cannabis strains (e.g. Skunk) that convert a lot of CBG into THC are low in CBD. Other strains (e.g. Charlotte's Web) convert most of the CBG into CBD and thus are low in THC. A secondary, less-expensive source of CBD exists in the stalks, leaves, and flowers of industrial hemp, which contains 15 percent CBD with only trace amounts of THC (0.3 percent). Finally, CBD can be produced by chemical synthesis. Most CBD sold today comes from industrial hemp and has nothing to do with marijuana.

CBD is available in a wide variety of products, including oils to be dripped beneath the tongue, capsules, creams to be rubbed on joints, tinctures, patches, gummy bears, liquid used for vaping, cosmetics (e.g. lip balm), pet treats, and even CBD-impregnated face masks. Non-users of marijuana are more likely to use CBD than marijuana users. Over 60 percent of CBD is used to treat a medical condition, primarily pain, anxiety, or depression.

Leaving the topic of how CBD works to be answered by professors and graduate students trying to make a name for themselves, the central questions most people have are "Is it safe?" and "Does it work?" What does science tell us about these important questions?

Safety can never be guaranteed with 100 percent certainty as there is no way to prove that something bad could never happen, but studies evaluating the safety of CBD in adults have generally been quite reassuring. Careful review of the medical literature finds that CBD's main side effects are minor and include tiredness, diarrhea, and changes in appetite and weight. No serious or rare reactions have been reported. The truth is that CBD has a better side-effect profile than many of the other drugs used to treat the conditions that CBD may benefit. Many benefits attributed to the THC in medical marijuana may be more due to CBD, and CBD lacks many of the side effects of THC, most notably getting high or becoming dependent. CBD has no street value as a drug of abuse. No one seeks treatment for CBD addiction because it does not exist. The World Health Organization has concluded that CBD has no potential for abuse or dependence.

Despite this generally clean bill of health for CBD, two cautions should be noted. Interactions between CBD and other medications have not been fully researched and are likely to emerge only as they arise and are reported. Because CBD is metabolized by a complex group of enzymes in the liver, it can potentially impact medications that are also broken down by the same enzymes. This includes 60 percent of the most common medications, from anti-epileptics to blood thinners and the commonplace statins used to reduce cholesterol. When CBD is introduced, it can interfere with the metabolism of other medications, often increasing their concentration and perhaps necessitating a reduction in their dose. Although CBD–drug interactions are common, they are not usually clinically important. Still, it is always recommended to inform your doctor if you are taking CBD so that its impact on prescribed medications can be monitored.

Second, CBD's safety has not been evaluated for children and fetuses. The impact CBD could have on developing brains may be quite different from its limited impact on mature brains. In a similar way, a strong storm can rip the buds off fruit trees, ruining the crop, but the same storm later in the season would do little harm to ripening fruit. Just because CBD is well tolerated by a pregnant woman is no guarantee that her unborn child's brain is also safe. Using CBD as a supplement to calm children may affect their brain development; we simply do not know. Advertisements claiming precise and proper dosing for children are not proof of safety. CBD should not be considered a wellness supplement, especially for children, as its impact on the brain is so widespread. It's better to find out why your child is anxious rather than blindly treating him or her with medication, and if medication is truly justified, it's better to seek the advice of someone trained in diagnosing and treating childhood anxiety. Caution is warranted.

Pain

As noted in the previous chapter, there is substantial scientific evidence that both THC and CBD (and especially the two together) reduce pain and inflammation. The analgesic and anti-inflammatory effects of cannabinoid stimulation are demonstrated by the interference of NSAIDs with an enzyme released by inflammation that breaks down cannabinoids. Thus, NSAIDs work in part by increasing anandamide and 2-AG. Our natural cannabinoids relieve pain, and adding CBD to the mix stimulates the ECS to produce analgesia by further increasing anandamide and 2-AG and changing the shape of cannabinoid receptors to modify their response to endocannabinoid transmitters.

There is evidence to suggest that states with legal medical cannabis have seen a reduction in opiate use. Anyone using chronic opiate treatment for pain should speak to their doctor and discuss adding CBD, or both CBD and THC, to see if their opiate dose can be reduced. The goal is to find the mixture of opiates and cannabinoids that gives maximum pain relief with minimum side effects, perhaps with special attention paid to avoiding clouded mental acuity. Avoiding feeling drugged or impaired is difficult when significant pain relief is required. For this reason, starting with CBD alone makes the most sense.

Anxiety

The first research indicating that CBD reduces anxiety came with the observation that giving CBD in conjunction with THC reduces the amount of anxiety THC can create. CBD alone does not appear to lower anxiety below an individual's normal baseline level, although research shows that CBD can reduce anxiety that has been elevated above normal levels. CBD successfully reduced signs of anxiety in rats challenged to navigate a maze of walkways elevated above water, which is obviously an anxiety-inducing situation. When humans are placed in anxiety-producing situations, such as taking a test that requires an unrehearsed speech or viewing pictures designed to make people anxious, CBD lowers their anxiety reaction. This reduction of "excess" anxiety can be objectively measured. The amygdala, which produces the fight or flight reactions, remains calmer when viewing the anxiety-inducing pictures if CBD has been administered. Perspiration on the palms, typically monitored in lie detector tests to indicate increased anxiety, is also reduced. CBD clearly decreases the elevation of anxiety above normal baseline levels that occurs with certain stressors and medical conditions. It does not appear to lower anxiety below its normal floor, distinguishing it from benzodiazepines like Valium and Xanax, which can continue lowering anxiety to levels of comfortable numbness, stupor, and eventually coma.

Up to 33 percent of the population suffers from an anxiety disorder at some point in their lifetime, including generalized anxiety, panic disorder, post-traumatic stress, social anxiety, and obsessive-compulsive disorders. Anxiety is a normal part of life and is even a useful emotion that can alert us to dangers and increase performance at critical times, but excessive anxiety can interfere with normal functioning and quality of life. Anti-anxiety medications, such as selective serotonin reuptake inhibitors (SSRIs, e.g. Prozac), benzodiazepines, and mood stabilizers like gabapentin, are not always effective treatments and each has its own side effects. SSRIs are notorious for reducing sexual performance. Benzodiazepines can be highly addictive and generate rebound anxiety when each dose wears off. While mood stabilizers are generally better tolerated, their benefit can be limited. The serious downsides of these medications invite the development of treatment with CBD or undiscovered CBD derivatives.

A final word of caution is needed. As with all medicinal treatments, their effectiveness is enhanced when accompanied by lifestyle changes. For example, statins taken to lower cholesterol are more effective when accompanied by dietary change and increased exercise. Likewise, medication for anxiety can be a critical part of a treatment plan, but its effectiveness is enhanced when patients are willing to do the hard work of changing behavior or seeing a psychotherapist for long enough to develop a healthier attitude and lifestyle.

Depression

Depression is the third most common reason people use CBD, but credible evidence that it is an effective treatment is lacking. Existing studies of CBD's impact on depression have produced very conflicting results. Even the most avid believers in CBD's treatment of depression rely almost exclusively on animal models – rats specifically bred for behaviors that resemble characteristics of human depression, such as lassitude, decreased mobility, and disinterest in novelty or sources of pleasure. There are limitations to studying CBD's impact on animal models of depression. Animal models can only measure outward, vegetative signs of depression, but have no access to the subjective, inner suffering characteristic of the condition, such as depressed mood, low self-esteem, or suicidality. In other words, scientific research has a very long way to go before animal studies offer any reliable evidence that CBD benefits depression.

Even searching the web only results in a few testimonials in which pain and anxiety accompany depression. It is easy to understand how life could be less depressing when your pain and anxiety are lessened, which CBD can do. Despite the lack of scientific evidence, marketers continue to claim that their CBD products relieve depression, emphasizing its lack of negative side effects compared with traditional medications. As one advocate mused, "Imagine a scenario where the world's most effective antidepressant is growing naturally all around us!" Unfortunately, this appears to be purely imagination at this point. While CBD is an effective medicine for many ailments, it becomes nothing more than snake oil when sold as a remedy for which there is no legitimate scientific evidence.

Marketers also promote cannabis products containing THC as treatment for depression. While it is true that many people feel an immediate improvement of their mood with THC, this is not proof that cannabis is a good treatment for depression. Cocaine likewise produces an immediate lifting of mood, but no one mistakes cocaine's euphoria as anything but a temporary, although often welcome, distraction from their underlying depressed mood. Chronic use of cocaine leads to addiction and profound depression upon withdrawal. Although at a far less intense degree, the same is true of chronic use of THC to alleviate depression. Chapters 10 and 11 explain the impact of too-frequent cannabis use.

Sleep

Beyond the three most common uses for CBD listed above, several ailments have received interesting preliminary support. In my own practice, I have frequently seen CBD taken as a sleep aid, but its effect on sleep seems to be hit or miss. One survey found that over 40 percent of people taking CBD experienced improved sleep. When it works, people love CBD because it doesn't have the "hangover" many get from traditional sleeping pills. When it doesn't work, which happens 60 percent of the time, no harm is done beyond the cost of the product and disappointment with the lack of benefit.

Research on CBD for sleep has found conflicting results, perhaps for two reasons. First, there is confusion about the correct dose to use. Mechoulam found that low doses (15 mg) interfere with sleep, while higher doses (160 mg) produce significantly better sleep. Unfortunately, 70 percent of CBD products have been found to mislabel their contents, so accurate dosing is difficult. Second, people participating in CBD sleep research have often not been well screened. Participants who have sleep that is disturbed by anxiety or pain are far more likely to receive benefit from CBD. Others with a primary sleep disorder may be less likely to receive benefit.

If this is confusing, there is one sure way to sort matters out. CBD is safe enough to try. Experiment with different doses to see what works best for you, or if it even works at all. Believe your own experience. I never doubt people who swear CBD helps them sleep better. Whether CBD is actually treating their anxiety and pain, treating a primary sleep disorder, or is just a good placebo is of little concern. If sleep is a problem, as it is for 80 percent of people at least once a week, give it a try. But do not become complacent and neglect exploring behavioral change as well. If you are trying to tolerate a higher level of anxiety than what is healthy for you, covering this problem up with CBD is nothing more than holding yourself together with baling wire and duct tape while delaying a final reckoning with an unhealthy lifestyle.

Jevon's experience of an initial benefit that soon faded is the most common experience my patients have reported. He was not harmed by the trial, and you probably will not be either. Don't blame yourself if it does not work, and do not let CBD or any other medication serve as a substitute for good sleep hygiene and a healthy lifestyle.

Psychotic Episodes and Schizophrenia

It is important to distinguish between the mental condition of psychosis and the disease of schizophrenia. The essential characteristic of psychosis is a loss of normal reality testing. When psychotic, an individual may have blatantly false beliefs (delusions, including paranoid delusions), may see and hear things others do not (hallucinations), and may speak incoherently with a flight of ideas that have no logical connection. When psychotic, individuals are generally unaware they are misperceiving reality. As a result, interactions with psychotic individuals can often be baffling, upsetting, and bizarre. The many causes of psychosis include medical conditions, extreme sleep deprivation, mental illness such as schizophrenia and bipolar disorder, medications, and drugs such as alcohol, stimulants, and cannabis. While nearly all healthy adults experience anxiety when given intravenous THC, 50 percent also develop psychotic symptoms, including paranoia. The level of anxiety experienced does not seem to be related to whether psychotic symptoms occur. THC-induced agitation and psychosis are reduced when CBD is given alongside the THC. Because the amount of THC and CBD are inversely related in the cannabis flower, states legalizing high-THC marijuana have reported an increase in emergency room visits for cannabis-induced acute psychosis. Fortunately, these bad trips generally resolve with only supportive care.

The brain disorder leading to schizophrenia is complex, and so is the impact of cannabinoids on this often-devastating illness. However, the fact that CBD reduces THC-induced psychosis raises the question of whether it might also benefit the treatment of schizophrenia. One certainty has been reached in the midst of these complexities: THC is one of the worst drugs for schizophrenics to use, and it may trigger, intensify, and even precipitate the disease. Studies now show that CBD not only protects against THC-induced psychosis but may possibly have a beneficial impact on some schizophrenic patients.

Schizophrenia strikes approximately 1 percent of the population, with an average onset during a person's late teens or early 20s. While the degenerative brain disorders discussed in Chapter 8 all have prominent physical symptoms, schizophrenia's impact is mostly mental. Although the exact cause of schizophrenia isn't known, genetics and brain chemistry are commonly believed to be contributing factors, and its effects are largely cognitive, emotional, and psychological. Psychiatrists divide symptoms into positive and negative groups. Positive symptoms include the *appearance* of behaviors not normally experienced, such as hallucinations, delusions, and "crazy talk," or language disconnected from the usual logic of cause and effect, and occasionally a tossed salad of unrelated words and ideas. Negative symptoms include the *absence* of behaviors that are normally present, such as blunted emotions, profound apathy, low social need, an inability to feel pleasure, and a general withdrawal from the world shared by the rest of us. Schizophrenia is a lifetime disorder with no known cure, although medication may reduce symptoms enough to permit 50 percent of sufferers to work and live independently within 10 years of their diagnosis. In the worst cases, patients become unreachable and incapable of caring for their food or shelter. Despite the public's general discomfort with psychotic behavior, schizophrenics are rarely violent.

Large-scale studies show that cannabis use increases the rate of schizophrenia in the general population. For example, among 45,000 Swedish army recruits followed for 15 years, those who used cannabis had a twofold increase in their rate of schizophrenia. While this association does not explain whether cannabis caused more schizophrenia or if those who were fated to develop schizophrenia were more likely to use cannabis, it is crucial to remember that THC alone can cause transient psychotic symptoms in laboratory settings. However, when people receive CBD before a high dose of THC, they develop less anxiety and have fewer psychosis-like behaviors. Outside the laboratory, users of cannabis flowers particularly high in THC (and therefore low in CBD) experience a fourfold increase in their rate of schizophrenia. Surveys of European cities demonstrated a higher rate of schizophrenia-like psychosis in areas where the THC content of locally available marijuana is higher. The conclusion these studies reach is that THC causes temporary psychosis and schizophrenia-like illness, while CBD modifies the negative effect of THC. The protective impact of CBD on THC is one reason public health experts worry about the increasingly popular, high-THC products sold in dispensaries today. Whether heavy cannabis use causes schizophrenia or whether it only further tips the balance against those who already have a genetic predisposition is still an unanswered question.

THC increases psychotic symptoms in people who are already schizophrenic, often to the point of decompensating them enough to require more frequent hospitalizations. It has even been shown that schizophrenics who use cannabis suffer more loss of brain volume than schizophrenics who abstain. It is clear that THC aggravates schizophrenia, should be avoided by anyone with this diagnosis, and should be used with great caution, if at all, by anyone with a family history of schizophrenia.

The relationship between CBD and schizophrenia is less clear. A double-blind study of schizophrenics divided patients into two groups: one group received CBD, and the other received a placebo. Both groups also received their usual antipsychotic medication. Six weeks later, clinicians rated those given CBD to have fewer symptoms and to be better functioning than those given the placebo. Only one well-controlled study has shown that CBD alone produces better results than antipsychotic medication in paranoid schizophrenia, one of the most difficult forms of schizophrenia to treat. These scattered results leave us currently unable to draw any final conclusions about CBD in the treatment of schizophrenia. The theory that CBD might be useful has some merit and seems attractive, but there is not yet enough good scientific evidence to recommend its use, only to recommend further research. Because CBD has very few side effects and an excellent safety record, we should expect that such studies will eventually be undertaken.

Epilepsy

The use of cannabis to treat epilepsy has a long history. However, only recently has CBD been tested and scientifically proven to be useful. In the 1970s, Brazilian scientists added CBD to anticonvulsant medication for a small number of patients with uncontrolled seizures. All but one improved significantly, and yet it took the development of a strain of cannabis with very high CBD called Charlotte's Web to produce enough interest to launch serious research in the USA. Charlotte's Web was promoted as a medication for two devastating forms of childhood epilepsy that are notoriously difficult to treat: Lennox–Gastaut and Dravet syndromes. Eventually, the FDA approved an effective CBD medication called Epidiolex for these childhood forms of epilepsy. An extract of cannabis produced by GW Pharmaceuticals, Epidiolex contains more than 99 percent CBD and less than 0.1 percent THC in a standardized dose.

The availability of Epidiolex enables further research. One study has already shown that adding CBD to standard anticonvulsant medication for adults and children with treatment-resistant epilepsy produces significant and sustained improvement. This study was not double-blind and did not include a placebo control, so confirmation of its findings is still needed. We can expect CBD to be a rapidly evolving story in the treatment of epilepsy for years to come.

Organ Transportation

Organs require quick transport to medical centers with the capacity to perform transplant surgery. As soon as a heart or kidney is removed from the body and placed in a cooler, its blood supply is interrupted and the tissue begins to deteriorate due to low oxygen levels. CBD's anti-inflammatory and antioxidant properties suggested a possible role in maintaining the viability of organs subjected to oxidative stress during transport. Studies soon showed that CBD provides the same benefits to organs harvested for transplantation that it provides to animals with a temporary blockage of blood supply to their heart or brain. Adding CBD to organ transport solutions protects the tissue and reduces organ rejection. In 2018, the FDA approved the addition of CBD to the solution organs are bathed in during transportation.

Retina Degeneration and Diabetic Blindness

Damage from oxygen deprivation and inflammation occurs for reasons other than the interruption of blood flow by clots, as happens during strokes and heart attacks. For example, diabetic retinopathy is the leading cause of blindness in Americans between 20 and 75 years old, affecting 12,000 annually. This major complication of diabetes results from damage to the blood vessels that supply oxygen to light-sensitive retina cells in the back of the eye. These light receptors connect to neurons that pass signals back to the brain's visual system. Light receptors die when diabetes constricts and inflames the blood vessels nourishing the retina. No visual signals are sent to the brain, and blindness results. Studies of diabetic retinopathy in mice have shown that CBD injections activate antioxidant defenses against vascular inflammation and degeneration of the light receptors. This does not guarantee that CBD will treat diabetic retinopathy in humans; clinical studies still have to be conducted. However, CBD's proven antioxidant and anti-inflammatory effects and its demonstrated benefit in animal studies of diabetic retinopathy are consistent with stroke and heart attack studies. This consistency adds to the rationale for undertaking careful studies in human diabetics. The advance of medical science is always slower than we want because funding is limited and all research must be guided by the same Hippocratic principle that governs physicians to first "do no harm."

Conclusion

"Buyer beware" applies to more than just financial purchases. It also warns us to be critical about any ideas we are "buying." Be very wary of anything touted as a panacea. There are no medical panaceas. Our hope, and sometimes our political convictions, tempt us to see panaceas where none exist. This is a normal, although avoidable, part of life. Almost every new medication begins as a wonder drug pushed along by its manufacturer's overpromising, only to fall to earth and into proper perspective once it bumps up against the public's experience. Penicillin was a wonder drug. We marveled at its ability to cure infections never before treatable. With time, we began to realize its true limits, its tendency to produce dangerous allergic reactions, and the ability of bacteria to develop resistance. While cannabis and cannabinoid-based medications, including CBD, have not yet reached their full potential, they will eventually fall into their proper perspective. Panacea, the Greek goddess of universal remedy, was just a myth born out of the hope to rise above human frailty.

It is entirely possible for cannabis to simultaneously be the basis for valuable medications backed by solid evidence, a fad, a snake-oil medicine naively or cynically sold as a panacea, and a substance of potential abuse when containing THC. I urge you to view fatuous CBD products such as lemon-lime-infused toothpicks, hair conditioner, hand sanitizer, and pet treats as novelty items. These products may be fun but should not be used to validate or denigrate medications for which there is good scientific evidence. And I urge you to measure hyperbolic, vague, and unsubstantiated health claims against the evidence provided by science.

Finally, do not be afraid to ask your doctors for their objective advice about cannabis. Insist on being given more than mere opinion. If your doctor does not know the basic facts about THC and CBD contained in this book, encourage them to become better informed.

10 WHEN CANNABINOID RECEPTORS DISAPPEAR

Randy was a middle-aged businessman who maintained a charming, although too often irresponsible, adolescent quality. His life had never reached its potential and his marriage was threatened. An intermittently regular cannabis user since college, he told me about recently scoring some wildly good marijuana. This was the mid-1990s, when new varieties of powerful sinsemilla cannabis flower were becoming available in San Francisco. After smoking it every day for a couple of weeks, he exhausted his supply and was unable to find any more. He began feeling more fidgety and physically restless than normal, and he felt constantly anxious and irritable. Persistent insomnia drained his energy and interest in work. Randy asked if he was developing a sleep disorder, or maybe an anxiety disorder, that needed medical treatment. He wondered if he was getting depressed.

When I asked him to tell me more about the marijuana he had been smoking recently, Randy enthusiastically praised its power to help him unwind from the day's stress and relax physically and emotionally. While he was using it, he had slept like a baby and his mood had generally been great. Unsurprisingly, he was eager to find more of what he called "the good stuff." He summed it up by saying, "It was fantastic. Nothing had ever gotten me that high before." He scoffed at my suggestion that his discomfort might be an aftereffect of having used such strong cannabis. After a couple of weeks of abstinence, his discomfort faded and he dismissed the episode as being unimportant.

I was unable to forget the consequences of Randy's brief period of using "the good stuff." It was clear that the physical relaxation, stress relief, calming, and ease falling asleep while using the strong cannabis flower were all due to above-normal activation of his CB1 receptors by large amounts of THC. His discomfort following the period of use appeared to be the direct opposite of being high. Instead of experiencing the elevated ECS tone he had when high, he was likely experiencing decreased ECS tone afterward. I had never seen this rebound from high to low tone happen so clearly. As I put his experience in context with the accumulating research, I gradually understood what had happened to Randy.

Receptor Downregulation: An Inconvenient Truth

Normal tone in the ECS requires a normal number of cannabinoid receptors. The number of CB1 receptors in the brain can be decreased in three ways: CB1 receptors can be eliminated altogether, they can be blocked, or they can be progressively reduced in number. I will examine each of these ways individually.

First, researchers have identified the gene for CB1 receptors and eliminated it in a strain of mice. These mice appear outwardly normal despite having absolutely no CB1 receptors. The primary point of interest is the increased mortality of the mice. Their life span is shorter than normal, but not for any single reason. The mice die for all the same reasons normal mice die. The best theory for this increased mortality is that, without CB1 receptors, they are unable to modulate physiological functions the way a properly working ECS does. They lack flexibility in responding to stress. Mice without CB1 receptors are like rigid oaks rather than flexible willows, susceptible to the battering of life's storms. A healthy ECS allows us to meet stress more flexibly, bending when necessary, rather than resisting change. As a result, CB1-deficient mice are damaged more by normal life stressors and die earlier. Although this animal model graphically illustrates the fundamental value of a healthy ECS, it does not correspond to any condition realistically related to human experience.

Second, the CB1 receptor blocker rimonabant has clearly demonstrated how the experience of lower endocannabinoid tone is the mirror image of high endocannabinoid tone. When animals are given THC for several days, elevating CB1 activity, and then given rimonabant, they are suddenly thrown into low CB1 activity. Instead of being less physically active and generally placid, the animals become restless, agitated, and easily provoked into aggressive behavior. No one has reported similar research with humans, but humans have been given rimonabant for weight loss. Even without first being primed with THC, rimonabant's reduction of ECS tone caused depression, insomnia, nausea, vomiting, diarrhea, and fatigue. Inactivating the ECS leaves all other neurotransmitter systems without the regulation the ECS provides through negative feedback as described in Chapter 3. We need our natural ECS to be working normally in order to feel well and maintain homeostasis. Lowering endocannabinoid tone below normal levels produces some of the same discomfort in people who stop the frequent use of cannabis, as Randy experienced when he ran out of his "good stuff," namely anxiety, depressed mood, restlessness, irritability, and insomnia.

Third, the frequent use of cannabis reduces the number of functioning CB1 receptors. Brain imaging shows as much as a 20 percent reduction (called downregulation) of receptors in the frontal cortex of regular users. Animal studies show that THC is the cause of this reduction of CB1 receptors. CBD alone does not trigger a reduction, but THC alone reduces CB1 receptors in some areas of the brain by as much as 60 percent after just 2 weeks of exposure.

THC's reduction of CB1 receptors is an important fly in the ointment that needs to be well managed by anyone using cannabis recreationally or medicinally. The phrase "fly in the ointment" comes from the Bible's book of Ecclesiastes and means a drawback to something valuable, especially a drawback that was not originally seen. In the case of cannabis, THC's powerful activation of cannabinoid receptors has the unintended consequence of downregulating those receptors. Before any readers jump to an unwarranted conclusion, I should add that this unintended consequence *can* be managed. If not understood and responded to properly, however, too-frequent or too-heavy use of cannabis products containing THC can cause negative side effects similar to those Randy experienced.

The concept of homeostasis, or the tendency toward maintaining equilibrium, is useful for understanding the potential drawbacks of cannabis. When THC occupies CB1 receptors, its powerful and long-lasting activation suppresses the amount of neurotransmitter released by neural systems throughout the brain much more than normally produced by anandamide and 2-AG. This extraordinary amount of negative feedback lasts for many hours of medical relief or recreational pleasure. Stimulating a level of negative feedback beyond normal physiological limits disturbs the brain's chemical balance and activates a homeostatic mechanism designed to return the brain to equilibrium. Neurons do this by downregulating the number of CB1 receptors available to be activated. With fewer CB1 receptors subjected to THC's abnormal level of activation, the total amount of negative feedback is reduced to a level closer to normal. Downregulation begins with even a single use of cannabis, pulling some CB1 receptors away from floating in the cell membrane and into the neuron's interior. Once sequestered inside the neuron, they are protected from THC's activation. The receptor returns to float in the membrane again, half outside the cell and half inside, soon after THC dissipates.

However, if cannabis is used again before all the CB1 receptors have been "upregulated," a deficit in CB1 receptors begins to accumulate. With continued, frequent use, CB1 receptors become progressively more downregulated to as much as 20 percent of normal in the cortex and 60 percent of normal in other areas of the brain. When receptors are kept inside the neuron too long, they begin being dismantled and the amino acids out of which they are built are used to construct other needed proteins. Overusing cannabis results in an ongoing CB1 deficit and dysregulation of the ECS. The relative lack of CB1 receptors begins to have the same effect as rimonabant's blocking action: below-normal activity in the ECS.

This process of downregulation is vital to understanding how to use cannabis safely. To illustrate the unintended consequences in the brain from too-frequent cannabis use due to THC's tendency to downregulate CB1 receptors, imagine an immensely successful marketing campaign at a major bank that rewards customers for using ATMs more frequently. A sudden rush of new customers increases the number of ATM transactions beyond the processing ability of the bank's central computers. All bank operations are slowed, customers experience long wait times, and the computer system begins making errors. The immediate fix is to shut down enough ATMs to ease the burden on the bank's computer system. Transaction processing returns to normal (homeostasis) as ATMs are taken out of service (downregulated). This analogy illustrates how downregulation mitigates the impact of abnormally intense activity, whether stimulated by THC activating CB1 receptors or by new customers visiting ATMs. Although normal function can be approximated, this new normal exists far from the equilibrium for which the system was designed.

In a similar way, when a cloud of THC molecules enters the lungs, crosses into the blood, and then travels to the brain, CB1 receptors are quickly superactivated, termed "super" because no natural behaviors ever activate CB1 receptors to this extent. The result is a higher order of magnitude of negative feedback experienced by neurons throughout the brain, especially in areas where CB1 receptors are most densely concentrated (e.g. amygdala, basal ganglia, hippocampus). As this occurs in the brain, a person is likely to relax physically and emotionally, feel his or her mood elevate, have their attention drawn to pleasing sensations as though seen for the first time, and experience the slower passing of time. With even the first use of cannabis, brain homeostatic mechanisms will begin downregulating CB1 receptors. Although any sense of feeling high or drug altered in any way is likely to have vanished by the next morning, CB1 receptors will not yet have fully returned to their normal level. Receptor downregulation takes a bit longer to resolve than the experience of being high lasts.

The subtle impact of receptor downregulation 24 hours after cannabis use was best demonstrated over three decades ago with professional airline pilots. In this intriguing study, the baseline performance of a group of experienced pilots was measured in a flight simulator. Then the pilots were given a joint to smoke. This study was conducted back in the 1980s, so it is likely that the marijuana used was considerably less potent than what is available today, perhaps as low as 3 percent THC, but the joint's dose and THC:CBD ratio were not measured. The next day, the pilots returned to repeat the flight simulator test. Although none were aware of any impairments or had any remaining sense of being high, they flew their virtual airplane toward the runway at higher or lower elevations than their baseline performance, landed less centered on the runway, and made significantly more adjustments to their flight path as they approached landing. Flying a plane is a highly complex task requiring intense concentration, sharpened fine motor control, and accurate hand–eye coordination. Each pilot's reactions to unexpected events in the simulation were slower and less organized than the day before. In a situation where strong crosswinds, downdrafts, or decreased visibility suddenly complicated the task, having used marijuana 24 hours previously would put a pilot at a clear disadvantage and endanger passengers.

CB1 receptor downregulation produces a condition called endocannabinoid dysregulation. With a single use of cannabis, endocannabinoid dysregulation negatively impacts the performance of highly complex tasks for at least 24 hours. Safety-sensitive professions, such as airplane pilots, air traffic controllers, crane operators, and surgeons, are most likely to experience negative consequences the next day. Receptor downregulation is soon reversed through upregulation, and it is unlikely that endocannabinoid dysregulation from a single use of cannabis lasts much more than 24 hours, although this is not known for sure, and differences among individuals undoubtedly exist.

A different picture develops when cannabis use is repeated before receptor upregulation is complete. This situation is especially likely to occur with daily use. Again, animals given THC daily for 2 weeks show reductions of CB1 receptors of 20–60 percent, depending on what areas of the brain are measured. Downregulation in humans who use cannabis regularly has been measured with sensitive brain imaging technology, and the studies found that the outer cortex of the brain has 20 percent fewer than normal active CB1 receptors in regular cannabis users. This reduction is especially prominent in the frontal areas of the cortex, where our most complex cognitive functions are produced, including abstract think-ing, planning, and judgment.

Fortunately, cannabinoid downregulation is largely reversible. The same brain imaging techniques have shown that total abstinence from cannabis use leads to complete, or nearly complete, upregulation within 4 weeks, with the bulk of upregulation occurring early in that window. In other words, regular cannabis use by adults does not fry the brain or cause permanent damage the way other drugs and alcohol can. I should stress that this is true for adults but not necessarily true if cannabis is used too early in adolescence, an important topic that is explored in Chapter 12.

The Experience of Downregulation

Research findings are fascinating, but it is not always clear how they are connected to our day-to-day reality. Exactly what is the relevance of endocannabinoid receptor down-regulation to the average cannabis user? What is the experience of cannabinoid downregulation?

When high-potency marijuana became available in the San Francisco area during the mid-1990s, patients began complaining of restlessness, anxiety, general discomfort, irritability, loss of appetite, and insomnia when they ran out of this new, more powerful pot. These complaints exactly paralleled reports of behavior seen in rats, cats, dogs, and monkeys who were given rimonabant after a couple of weeks of daily THC exposure. All these species experienced physical restlessness with "wet dog shakes," increased signs of anxiety, aggression, lack of appetite, and insomnia. Humans are animals too, but can describe the subjective experience of their endocannabinoid dysregula-tion. Patients were uncomfortable, although they never suffered as much as those abstaining from most other drugs. Their discomfort ranged between that reported by people deprived of their morning coffee and smokers denied their cigarettes (see Chapter 11 for more detail). Many found that the single best way to relieve their restlessness, anxiety, irritability, and insomnia was to resume cannabis use. THC's strong stimulation of the remaining CB1 receptors approximated the impact of anandamide and 2-AG's stimulation of a normal number of receptors, and they felt more like their normal selves.

Five Signs of Using Cannabis Too Frequently

Newton's physical law – for every action there is an equal and opposite reaction – is also true in the drug world. What goes up must come down and what goes down must come up. Drug withdrawal is roughly the mirror image of the drug's effect. The drowsy, pain-free dreaminess of an opiate high is mirrored in withdrawal by excruciating emotional and physical discomfort and nervous excitement. The high energy and elevated mood of stimulants are mirrored in withdrawal by profound lethargy and depression. The characteristics of a cannabis high that stand out for many people are physical relaxation, emotional calming, freshened and vivified sensations, increased appetite (the "munchies"), and ease of falling asleep. While these characteristics do not describe everything people treasure about the cannabis experience, they are important for understanding the withdrawal that mirrors a cannabis high.

When the regular use of cannabis is stopped, and even when very heavy users wake in the morning after several hours of no use during sleep, they may experience the unpleasant signs of deficient endocannabinoid tone. The five signs of using cannabis too frequently are:

1. Physical restlessness and feeling fidgety, often worse when trying to fall asleep.
2. Anxiety and irritability.

3. Boredom (the opposite of novel, freshened, and inten-
    sified sensations).
4. Loss of appetite.
5. Insomnia.

There is, of course, an immediate antidote: cannabis.
Because regular THC stimulation of the ECS has downregulated receptors, when THC activation of the remaining
receptors wanes, the normal amount of less potent,
shorter-acting anandamide and 2-AG cannot find enough
remaining receptors to match THC's more powerful stimulation. The cannabinoid tone in the ECS goes from being
higher than normal to lower than normal. This can be
temporarily rectified by adding back some THC. Although
this temporarily returns endocannabinoid tone to an
approximation of normal or above, it also promotes
further receptor downregulation. This is a Band-Aid, not
a long-term solution. A person in this situation has become
dependent on the presence of THC to feel more or less
normal. While people may consider this to be the essence
of addiction, it is really only one aspect, and is not even the
core facet of addiction. That topic will be covered in
Chapter 11.

Knowing the five signs of cannabinoid downregulation
is the key to using cannabis safely. These signs indicate
the presence of endocannabinoid dysregulation that
results from using cannabis too frequently. Everyone's
brain has its own unique capacity to tolerate the receptor-
downregulating impact of THC, just as it has its own
unique capacity to upregulate. There are no universal
standards or rules for how often or how much cannabis is
safe. Each individual has to monitor their own risk potential.
The five signs can provide the evidence each person needs
to recognize when the frequency and amount of their
cannabis use is outstripping their brain's capacity to maintain a normal, healthy balance. As physical and mental
wellness depend on a well-balanced ECS, a subtle decline in

wellness creeps in when endocannabinoid tone is deficient. Noticing the gradual appearance of increased restlessness, anxiety/irritability, boredom, loss of appetite, and insomnia depends on knowing these signs well enough to be on the lookout for them. Seeing the warning signs in yourself requires a high level of rigorous self-awareness and honesty. Others close to you may perceive these changes and understand their connection to cannabis before you do.

Why is it so difficult to notice cannabis-induced signs of endocannabinoid dysregulation in yourself? Perhaps the main reason is that cannabis use so clearly reverses these signs, at least temporarily. Cannabis quells restlessness, calms anxiety and irritability, makes everything more vivid and interesting, returns appetite, and aids sleep. What's not to like about that? The natural conclusion, even the accurate conclusion from a Cannabis Culture perspective, is that cannabis is a powerful medicine for what ails you. Randy latched onto this conclusion and consulted with his internist in an effort to diagnose what he believed were his underlying conditions. As he never mentioned his cannabis use to other doctors and they never asked, Randy underwent a bevy of laboratory tests and was prescribed several medications in a vain effort to correct his presumptive anxiety and sleep disorders. While it is true that cannabinoid-based medicines can be powerful, as outlined in Chapters 7–9, its reversal of the five signs of too-frequent cannabis use is a different thing. Cannabis-induced endocannabinoid dysregulation is not a primary disease in and of itself. When using cannabis too frequently leads to increased anxiety when the high is gone, this does not mean you have an anxiety disorder. When using cannabis too frequently leads to insomnia, this does not mean you have a sleep disorder. It means you have used cannabis enough to alter your brain beyond the period of being high. These signs mean you have been using cannabis to the point that the number of cannabin-oid receptors is depressed and will remain so until you have strung together enough days of total abstinence to allow your brain to upregulate receptors to their normal number. Chapter 6 described how members of Cannabis Culture who use cannabis primarily for spiritual purposes are clearly aware of the subtlest effects of endocannabin-oid dysregulation and have offered their own advice for using the drug most effectively.

Of course, you might have an anxiety or sleep disorder separate from your cannabis use. In that case, your under-lying disorder needs to be fully evaluated, properly diag-nosed, and effectively treated with the standard of care. None of us can accomplish this objectively on our own. Professional help should be sought, and the first test that should be administered is a period of abstinence long enough to assess your level of anxiety or insomnia separate from cannabis. The length of abstinence should be a minimum of 6 weeks, but preferably 3 months, depend-ing on the amount and length of use. If you are unable to successfully accomplish the required abstinence, careful consideration should be given to whether addiction has taken deeper root than endocannabinoid dysregulation alone can explain. In this case, a qualified addiction medi-cine specialist should be consulted.

In contrast, when people are fully aware of the five signs of using cannabis too frequently before initiating use, these signs can contribute to their safety. Mere awareness that there is a downside to too-frequent use disabuses people of the delusion that cannabis is entirely safe simply because it is organic. Knowing the signs to watch for enables people to recognize them earlier and at more subtle levels. When we pick up a pharmaceutical medica-tion at the drug store, we are warned that it can cause insomnia or diarrhea, for example, if our body is sensitive to it. It is ridiculous to think that anyone selling cannabis to you illegally would inform you of potential side effects, but it should be expected that legal sales should provide a brief, clear, written description of signs that cannabis use is exceeding safe limits. Even if your budista is less than candid about potential side effects, public health policy should require posting the signs of overuse and including written information describing them with your purchase. These steps would help the public be more likely to recognize the significance of their warning signs.

Such public health measures do not exist for the alcohol industry, perhaps because most people already know that tremors and sweating, for example, are signs of alcohol withdrawal, although they may be less aware that anxiety, irritability, and insomnia are also signs. Unfortunately, the alcohol industry is likely to strenuously resist any public health requirement to distribute such information. Big Alcohol is simply too powerful, too politically influential, and too well integrated into our cultural fabric to be forced into more responsible behavior. The cannabis industry is also growing rapidly in power and has already been integrated into large segments of our culture. Soon, Big Marijuana will become too impervious to regulation, if it is not already, to be required to contribute to public health education. Only time will tell. Meanwhile, the vast majority of people are currently unaware of even these five basic signs. Public health officials need to continue working toward increasing the public's scientific literacy about cannabis. The goal is safe use, and knowledge is our only weapon.

Diversions Versus Solutions

Knowledge of the five signs of downregulated cannabinoid receptors is useful, but, unfortunately, it is no guarantee that cannabis will be used safely. It is difficult to be rigorously honest about the appearance of warning signs because of the pleasure cannabis brings. This is true of many other pleasures as well. Food, for example, is a great pleasure for many people. There are clear, visible signs when we are eating too frequently or too much. Our clothes feel tight or need to be replaced with larger sizes. The numbers on our scale keep increasing. We know we are overweight, but we often don't pay attention to it beyond clucking at our tight pants and the rising numbers on the scale. Then, when a donut catches our attention, especially our favorite chocolate-covered cake donut, we give little thought to what we know. The cognitive dissonance created by watching ourselves do something that we know has negative consequences is too uncomfortable to focus on for long. We deny ourselves full awareness of what we are doing in order not to deny ourselves the donut, just this one time. Any number of rationalizations are trotted out. We made a healthier choice for breakfast, for example. Or the morning's work has been stressful. Or a tense meeting is scheduled for later in the day. Or we just completed an important task. Our psychology is well practiced at protecting our pleasures. If others try to help protect us against ourselves, we usually become defensive enough to shut down the conversation or remorseful enough to gain their forbearance. As important as they are, public health warnings are particularly easy to gloss over after we've seen them several times.

Finally, as a psychiatrist with a career-long fascination with alcohol and other drug use, I am familiar with many people's tendency to take the easy way out of discomfort. As coronavirus fatigue made social isolation increasingly difficult, alcohol and cannabis use continued to rise. The cannabis industry began reporting record profits. Any chemical that quickly and reliably alters our consciousness and provides an escape is seductive. I am not referring to addiction, but rather the idea of substituting a short-term diversion for a long-term solution. When this strategy becomes a pattern, it has a mounting impact on the richness of satisfaction with, and quality of, our life. It is common for the constant tensions and uncertainties of modern life to exhaust our resources at the end of the day and over the years. A beer or glass of wine, or two, works to relax our brow. So too does a bit of cannabis, whether smoked or chewed as a gummy bear. Relaxation and finding distance from our troubles is such a fond and necessary pleasure. It prepares us to suit up again the next day and keep on truckin'. When this needed "hole in the day" is found too frequently by ingesting a chemical, we avoid developing the psychological tools needed to achieve the same solace. Better living through chemistry becomes a substitute for doing the hard work of making the changes in attitude or lifestyle that would protect us from suffering the level of stress our current life creates. Short-term diversions instead of long-term solutions. An evening of using medically prescribed tranquilizers or other commercially available substances to become comfortably numb, if done too frequently, can become another and another in a long string of evenings that lead to psychological stagnation. This is not to argue against the occasional use of chemistry to ease the discomforts and unpleasantries of life. Rather, it is an expression of concern when this strategy becomes too habitual or the sole tactic for tolerating stress. Self-prescribed chemical diversions almost never lead to the internal psychological changes needed for positive growth. Instead, they often permit people to tolerate problematic situations that ought to be changed. Cannabis can be misused as a short-term diversion just as easily as any other chemical. Unless we continue growing and maturing psychologically, we risk missing the deepest rewards life has to offer.

Conclusion

The bottom line is simple: if you choose to use cannabis, you will maximize your pleasure if you follow the public health slogan to "Know Your Limits." Understanding and paying attention to the five signs of overuse presented in this chapter will provide a helpful guide for using cannabis safely.

11 WHEN ADDICTION HIJACKS THE BRAIN'S REWARD SYSTEM

Christopher passed up opportunities to try cannabis until the summer before 11th grade. He hadn't wanted to smoke anything because it might jeopardize his very successful soccer career, and he hated watching his father's alcoholism throw the family into turmoil. As soon as he tried a joint at a party, he immediately enjoyed how "clean" it was compared with his father's drinking – no angry outbursts, no messy vomiting, and no miserable hangover. He went to another party the next weekend and left it with a bag of weed and rolling papers. He got stoned at home every day for the rest of the summer to amuse himself, better able to ignore and feel superior to his father.

Christopher intended to stop using as soon as the new school year started, but he didn't for a long list of reasons – his courses were not interesting, several teachers were jerks, and he liked how his mind tumbled over endless topics as if he were looking through a kaleidoscope. His grades began to suffer. He cared, but not enough to stop, choosing to get stoned whenever he could. He told himself he would stop when soccer season began. He tried, but he suffered from terrible insomnia and lacked energy at practice. His coach was disappointed that Christopher started the season out of condition. Christopher allowed himself to smoke just a little to get some sleep and pushed himself to get back in shape. Then an Achilles injury sidelined him. When his coach heard of his star player's marijuana use and kicked him off the team in disgust, Christopher returned to smoking daily to soothe his disappointment before deciding he *wasn't really interested in soccer anymore. He settled into a comforting romance with Mary Jane, his favorite term for marijuana, even vaping THC between classes.*

The previous chapter explored the role of cannabis-induced downregulation of CB1 receptors in producing withdrawal symptoms when cannabis use is reduced or discontinued. The five signs of using cannabis too frequently are the most easily observable withdrawal symptoms. Many readers are likely to see these symptoms as proof that cannabis is addictive. I would contend that these symptoms are only partial evidence of addiction and do not strike directly at the deepest core of the addictive process. I tried to describe how most people's reactions to endocannabinoid dysregulation are quite similar to how we respond to a wide variety of unpleasantries unrelated to cannabis. For example, many people struggle with food and being overweight, and they use the same strategies of rationalization, minimization, and denial of the problem to kick the can down the road. These mental gymnastics are obvious when a person who wants to lose weight finds reason in the moment to eat a donut for pleasure and not out of essential hunger. The same mental processes take place in people confronting the unpleasantries of cannabis withdrawal. In other words, it is easy to understand how people might ignore or misinterpret the subtle signs of cannabis withdrawal and continue using.

Hijacking the Brain

Although the phrase "hijack the brain," used to describe what happens when a drug activates the deeper core of addiction, may strike some as overly dramatic or inflammatory, the phrase serves an important purpose. To be "hijacked" necessarily implies something involuntary. No one chooses to be the victim of a car hijacking or to become addicted to a drug that hijacks their brain. Hijacking is something that happens to you outside your will, and it can change the course of your life temporarily, or even permanently.

A little history will set the stage for understanding how drugs of addiction hijack the brain. Back in the early 1950s, two Canadian researchers, James Olds and Peter Milner, were investigating a small collection of neurons called the nucleus accumbens. In the search to discover the function of these neurons, Olds and Milner placed an electrode into the nucleus accumbens of rats and permitted them to activate the electrode by pressing a lever. They watched as rats continued pressing the lever to the point of exhaustion, preferring direct stimulation of the nucleus accumbens over even food and water. The young researchers had identified the primary reward center of the brain.

We now know that evolution has developed a mechanism for increasing reward, and therefore motivation, for many essential survival behaviors such as eating, exercise, and sexual activity. When one of these behaviors happens, the level of dopamine increases in the reward center. Dopamine is the chemical of reward. As humans tend to enjoy eating and especially sex, the nucleus accumbens has also been called the pleasure center, although it might more objectively be called the "repeat center." Any activity that leads to increased dopamine in the nucleus accumbens is an activity that is likely to be repeated.

We now know that all drugs of addiction, from caffeine to tobacco, alcohol, opiates, cocaine, and amphetamines, raise the level of dopamine in the reward center. THC also increases dopamine in the reward center. These drugs can raise dopamine levels as much as ten times higher than any natural behaviors, such as eating and sex. When any drug, including THC, chronically maintains supernormal levels of dopamine in the reward center, the very structure and number of neurons in the center change. The result is that the motivation to consume the drug is increased, often to the detriment of motivation for other activities. We become the rat that forsakes food for the rewarding lever.

Chemical alteration of a person's motivation explains the hijacking of the brain that lies at the deepest core of addiction. Not everyone's reward center is equally suscep-tible to being hijacked, probably for genetic reasons, so people with a strong family history of addiction need to be more careful with the use of addictive substances. Christopher was not careful, and his family's tendency toward addiction primed him to be susceptible to depen-dence as well. His genetic predisposition to addiction likely played a role in how cannabis hijacked his brain so quickly.

Another perspective on the core of addiction is to understand the interesting difference between liking and wanting. This difference is illustrated by offering rats two bottles of water, one bottle also containing sugar and the other containing cocaine. Rats gravitate toward the sugar water. Rats "like" sugar water more than cocaine water. However, something very interesting happens if only sugar or only cocaine water is offered and then the supply is interrupted. Rats that are no longer able to obtain sips of sugar water visit the bottle less often and soon stop trying to drink altogether. But rats no longer able to obtain cocaine water continually revisit the bottle. In fact, they work harder to regain access to the cocaine. Rats "want" cocaine more than they "want" sugar. The difference is explained by cocaine's ability to raise dopamine levels in the reward center higher than sugar can. As a result, the motivation for finding and consuming cocaine is far greater than the motivation to obtain sugar. This chemi-cally induced bending of motivation lies at the core of addiction. Christopher wanted cannabis more than he wanted soccer.

Signs of Addiction

Current medical understanding of the potential for cannabis addiction comes from the work of Alan Budney, a professor at Dartmouth's School of Medicine. He offers four lines of evidence supporting the addictive potential of cannabis. The first, outlined above, is the release of supernormal levels of dopamine in the reward center, which is the essential element in all addictive substances. The second line of evidence is the similarity of symptoms seen in a wide variety of animal species when thrust into cannabis withdrawal by replacing daily THC intake with rimonabant. The third line of evidence is self-reported symptoms of withdrawal in humans that parallel other animals' withdrawal symptoms. And the fourth line of evidence is the consistency of worldwide surveys finding that approximately one in ten cannabis users over the age of 18 develops at least minimal withdrawal upon abstinence from frequent cannabis use.

One of Budney's most illuminating studies compared the intensity of withdrawal symptoms between tobacco and cannabis. He asked people withdrawing from each to rate the intensity of a wide range of symptoms, including irritability, restlessness, sleep difficulties, and aggression. Both groups rated the same levels of intensity for each of these withdrawal symptoms (Figure 11.1). Appetite differed for the two different drugs, with increased appetite in tobacco withdrawal and decreased appetite in cannabis withdrawal. Cravings are experienced more intensely in tobacco withdrawal, probably because people smoke a cigarette far more often in a day than a joint, so tobacco is associated with far more events that can stimulate craving – meals, phone calls, bathroom breaks, etc. The bottom line is that cannabis withdrawal is no more medically important than tobacco withdrawal. No one visits the ER with medically important symptoms from cannabis

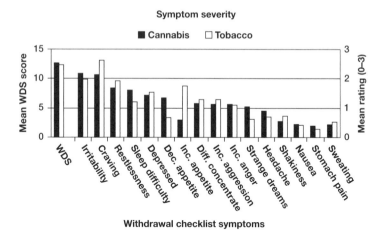

Figure 11.1 Tobacco versus cannabis withdrawal symptoms. Severity scores on the Withdrawal Discomfort Scale (WDS, vertical axis) and individual symptoms on the Withdrawal Symptom Checklist (horizontal axis) are shown. Asterisks indicate a significant difference after controlling for age, gender, race and Global Symptom Index scores.

withdrawal. The most common consequence of cannabis withdrawal is the same as seen in tobacco withdrawal: relapse. Absolutely nothing stops the discomfort of either withdrawal faster or more completely than restarting use. A simple solution to an aggravating problem.

The formal medical name for cannabis addiction is cannabis use disorder (CUD). The criteria for this diagnosis are built on Budney's organization of research data into a framework containing signs and symptoms from both THC's dysregulation of the ECS and its impact on the reward center. The following observable signs are the criteria for CUD in psychiatry's *Diagnostic and Statistical Manual of Mental Disorders, Fifth Edition* (DSM-5):

1. Use of cannabis for at least a 1-year period with the presence of at least two of the following symptoms, accompanied by significant impairment of functioning and distress.

2. Difficulty containing use of cannabis – the drug is used in larger amounts and over a longer period than intended.
3. Repeated failed efforts to discontinue or reduce the amount of cannabis that is used.
4. An inordinate amount of time is occupied acquiring, using, or recovering from the effects of cannabis.
5. Cravings or desires to use cannabis. This can include intrusive thoughts and images, dreams about cannabis, or olfactory perceptions of the smell of cannabis due to preoccupation with the drug.
6. Continued use of cannabis despite adverse consequences from its use, such as criminal charges, ultimatums of abandonment from spouse/partner/ friends, and poor productivity.
7. Other important activities in life, such as work, school, hygiene, and responsibility to family and friends, are superseded by the desire to use cannabis.
8. Cannabis is used in contexts that are potentially dangerous, such as operating a motor vehicle.
9. Use of cannabis continues despite awareness of physical or psychological problems attributed to use, e.g. anergia, amotivation, chronic cough.
10. Tolerance to cannabis, as defined by progressively larger amounts of cannabis needed to obtain the psychoactive effect experienced when use first commenced, or noticeably reduced effect of use of the same amount of cannabis.
11. Withdrawal, defined as the typical withdrawal syndrome associated with cannabis, or cannabis is used to prevent withdrawal symptoms.

The symptoms of the "typical withdrawal syndrome associated with cannabis" referred to in criterion 11 were identified by Budney as the following:

• Irritability, anger, or increased aggression.
• Nervousness or anxiety.

- Sleep difficulty (insomnia).
- Decreased appetite or weight loss.
- Restlessness.
- Depressed mood.
- At least one physical symptom causing significant discomfort (stomach pain, shakiness/tremors, sweating, fever, chills, headache).

The fact that cannabis meets the essential element for addiction by increasing dopamine in the reward center and the fact that reproducible symptoms of withdrawal can be described tells us that people can *potentially* become dependent on cannabis. However, these facts do not tell us how addictive cannabis is or why some people become addicted to it and others do not.

Addictive potential is measured by counting the number of people who ever try a drug once and then later meet the criteria used for diagnosing dependence. The most addictive recreational drug has always been legal: tobacco (nicotine). Thirty-two percent of people who ever try tobacco eventually become addicted. Surprisingly, only 23 percent of those who ever try heroin become addicted. Approximately 15 percent of those who ever try alcohol become addicted, and as many as 10 percent of individuals who ever experience cannabis as an adult become addicted at some point in their lives. The earlier in adolescence a teen begins any drug, including cannabis, the higher the risk of addiction.

Causes of Addiction

Who becomes dependent depends on many factors. Heredity is probably the most important influence, but it is hardly determinative. It has long been clear that drug addiction runs in families; this is especially obvious with alcoholism. When alcoholics are flagged on family trees, it is stunning to see the clustering that occurs in some family lines that is nearly absent in others. What genes are passed down to increase the likelihood that descendants will become alcoholic? There is no single alcoholism gene; it is a polygenetic disease, with multiple genes each adding their own particular influence. When the genetic dice are rolled by the randomness of which sperm fertilizes which egg, an individual is created with more or less tendency toward addiction. Some genes increase an individual's tendency to be attracted to novelty and risk-taking. Other genes produce a more cautious person more likely to draw back from novelty and minimize risk. Some genes amplify the amount of dopamine released in the reward center in response to any drug, while other genes reduce the level of dopamine release. The roll of the genetic dice is not fair. Each individual is left to figure out their own tolerance for drug usage, whether prescription, over the counter, or under the table. Unfortunately, some people need to figure this out when they're still quite young, well before their brains, minds, and personalities are fully developed. We are sometimes called upon to understand events affecting our health and lives before we have developed the capacity to comprehend such complexities.

What proof do we have that heredity is responsible for grandparents and parents (indeed, all of our ancestors) passing the tendency toward addiction down to the next generation? The answer to this important question is two-fold. The first clue comes from studies of twins born to alcoholic parents. The rate of alcoholism is the same in each sibling, even when one twin is adopted and raised by a non-alcoholic parent. Conversely, when one twin from non-alcoholic parents is raised in a family with an alcoholic parent, the rate of alcoholism is the same as the twin remaining with non-alcoholic parents. Other studies show that sons of alcoholic fathers respond differently, both physically and psychologically, to their first exposure to alcohol. Physical differences, such as amount of body sway and hormonal responses to alcohol, are unlikely to be learned behaviors. Genetic transmission is the most likely explanation for why such tendencies are repeated in the next generation. Nature has more influence than nurture when it comes to a brain's fundamental response to psychoactive drugs.

As powerful as heredity is, genetics are not the only push toward addiction. Poverty, nutritional deficits, exposure to violence, and countless other stresses can also increase future drug and alcohol abuse. Those who lack the personality traits and life experiences that create resilience are more likely to be attracted to the diversions and balm of drug use. There may be no stronger road to addiction than hopelessness, a trait that can pervade the culture in which one is fated to be born. Without a loving and nurturing adult to protect us against these stresses, it can be easy to be overwhelmed and swept toward whatever immediate relief presents itself. Condemnation of anyone for becoming drug dependent is a sign of arrogance and personal insecurity that results in the need to denigrate others to support one's own self-esteem by comparison.

Keeping Cannabis Dependence in Perspective

Contrary to the conventional wisdom among addiction treatment specialists that drug dependence is a lifelong disorder, the majority of people who meet the criteria for cannabis dependence do not remain dependent for their entire life. Chapter 12 will detail how most adolescents who become addicted eventually reduce or stop their cannabis use after a period of being dependent. The amount of damage done by a period of addiction depends significantly on when in a person's life they used cannabis to excess. If the period of dependence happens early in life, it can interfere with one's education in ways that more severely limit future career opportunities.

However, the vast majority of adults who have ever used cannabis, nine out of ten, use cannabis safely enough to avoid dependence. They never experience withdrawal symptoms. Of the few who do meet the criteria for CUD, the vast majority experience only a few symptoms of receptor downregulation and endocannabinoid dysregulation. Only after the reward center has been affected by chemical and structural changes do many of the more traditional signs of a deeper addictive process occur. When that happens, one's life begins being oriented more and more toward cannabis use, and the motivation to engage in other activities diminishes. Life begins revolving around cannabis as its central organizing principle. Environmental cues and reminders of cannabis attract more attention. Cannabis use becomes a higher priority than other activities because a person experiences the most reward from cannabis. Reward is not a cognitive process, but rather a basic feeling, a direct experience. As the attachment to cannabis increases, a greater sense of urgency and importance surrounds its use. These feelings are no longer an expression of one's psychology but rather stem from the direct result of THC's impact on brain structures that determine which experiences are rewarded, and therefore repeated. Addiction is unbidden, an unintended consequence of drug use.

Cannabis Alters Motivation

A fascinating experiment demonstrated THC's gradual hijacking of the reward system over 4 years of cannabis use. Motivation depends on the anticipation of reward. Participants in the study were given a menial computer task that required a response when specific stimuli appeared on the screen. The more accurately they performed the task, the greater the monetary reward would be when finished. Functional magnetic resonance imaging (fMRI) measured activity in the reward center during the computer task. At age 20, cannabis users and non-users both showed the same level of activity in the reward center in anticipation of a delayed monetary reward. However, by ages 22 and 24, the amount of activity in the reward center reflected the amount of cannabis used. The more an individual was using cannabis, the less activity occurred in the reward center in anticipation of a monetary reward. Although multiple explanations for this change can be proposed, researchers concluded that THC was gradually blunting the reward system's response to non-cannabis stimuli. The motivation for things not related to cannabis had declined. Cannabis had increasingly become the most important and desired reward. To what degree was this due to changes in their psychology or their brain? If they declared that money was not as important to them as it once was, would this have been because they had grown in wisdom or because their psychology had been dragged into alignment with the changes in their brain? Had their brain changed in response to wisdom conferred on them by their experience with cannabis, or had their psychology rationalized motivations altered by physical changes in the brain?

These questions present quite a conundrum. People in the Cannabis Culture see the answers as self-evident, while people looking through a scientific lens see a different set of answers. This is precisely the moment when laboratory animal studies become most valuable. When a wide range of different animal species are administered THC, increased levels of dopamine and structural changes occur in their nucleus accumbens. These changes to their reward system happen for purely physical reasons. No reference to their psychology, their experience of reward or pleasure, or an increase in wisdom needs to be cited to explain the brain changes. Furthermore, when the rats deprived of cocaine water worked harder to find another sip (i.e. were more motivated) than rats deprived of sugar water, this occurred because the cocaine had hijacked their reward system in a purely physical way. These animal experiments tilt the explanation of why cannabis use led to less activity in the reward system in anticipation of monetary reward toward physical changes in brain structure rather than psychological changes in perspective.

Rebellion Against Cannabis Addiction

It is difficult to know the extent to which the public accepts that cannabis addiction is real. Many are unsure, confused by their own benign experience and misinformation circulating on the Internet. Many others accept the reality of addiction but exaggerate its frequency and importance, and some minimize or deny the very possibility of cannabis addiction as government propaganda.

The reasons people are reluctant to acknowledge the possibility, or outright deny, that cannabis can be addictive are both personal and systemic. Denial of addiction is extremely common in people who are addicted themselves, or fear they may be addicted, to any drug they have integrated into their life. Addicts routinely defend their right to use their drug of choice, failing to realize that addiction has nothing to do with civil or personal rights. Whether an individual is addicted to any given drug has nothing to do with their right to consume that drug, although it often does have a lot to do with the wisdom of continuing to use it. People do not like having the wisdom of their choices challenged, whether by a partner, the law, a medical expert, or reality itself. They often develop elaborate, clever, and seemingly rational defenses of their choices. In the end, addiction is about physical changes to the brain that cause observable changes in behavior induced by frequent use of a drug. The criteria for diagnosing CUD are as objective and non-judgmental as medical experts can make them. When applied fairly, these criteria are a valuable tool for assessing whether an individual has reached a level of cannabis use that is harmful to themselves and others (i.e. whether they have become dependent on cannabis). Denial that cannabis can be addictive does not make addiction less real.

Many in the Cannabis Culture who are not addicted nevertheless resist accepting the possibility of cannabis addiction, and many outright deny the prospect. During the birth of Cannabis Culture among the dominant white culture of the 1960s, marijuana contained little more than 3 percent THC. Obtaining hash that was higher in THC was rare for most users. As a result, signs of endocannabinoid dysregulation and withdrawal were not often seen at that time, cannabinoid receptors had not yet been discovered, and cannabis addiction was not formally recognized by medicine. From the beginning, Cannabis Culture contained a deep current of rebellion against the traditional American mores of the buttoned-down 1950s, against the war in Vietnam, and against the authority of older generations in general. Such rebellion continues today, as members of the Cannabis Culture revolt against the War on Drugs, fight for full legalization of cannabis, and chastise the medical community for failing to explore the potential benefits of cannabis-based medication more earnestly.

Unfortunately, this rebellious streak has tolerated a lot of anti-scientific nonsense. Cannabis advocates can be heard declaring that all cannabis use is medicinal, that cannabis is 100 percent safe because it is natural, and that warnings about cannabis being addictive are politically motivated lies. These claims turn a blind eye to the fact that all medicines have potential side effects. They conflate natural and organic with safety, even though no one would feel safe eating death cap mushrooms simply because they grow naturally.

I have also heard members of the Cannabis Culture claim that THC is safer than nicotine because it is natural, as though tobacco isn't also a natural part of the botanical world. In defense of THC's safety, they offer that it is a cannabinoid and the brain contains natural cannabinoids and cannabinoid receptors. The argument that nicotine is not naturally found in the body ignores several important facts. First, THC is not naturally found in the body. It is as alien to our body as nicotine. The receptors activated by THC are designed for anandamide and 2-AG, not for THC. The only reason anandamide and 2-AG are called cannabinoids is because they activate receptors that were named after the synthetic cannabinoid molecules used to discover them. Nicotine was also used to discover "nicotinic receptors" that were designed by evolution to respond to neurotransmitters naturally found in the body. The fact that nicotine activates a receptor named after it for historical reasons does not make nicotine natural to our bodies. All of these confusions and misrepresentations of scientific fact merely serve to defend cannabis against anything that Cannabis Culture fears might denigrate its importance or give reason for caution in its sale and use.

The Gateway Theory and the Stigma of Addiction

Cannabis Culture is allergic to the idea that their drug could have addictive qualities because they seek to defend against restrictions on its availability and hope to avoid the stigma associated with the word addiction. The stain of addiction is further enhanced by the belief that cannabis is a gateway drug. Because nearly everyone who uses a hard drug later in life also used cannabis at an earlier age, people have associated cannabis use with more serious and destructive drug use. This association leads people to believe that cannabis is the cause of later hard-drug use. They are confusing association with cause, a common misconception that impairs science literacy. Almost everyone who has an automobile accident has ridden a bicycle earlier in their life, but it would be absurd to claim that riding a bike leads to car accidents, despite a nearly 100 percent association between the two. The fact that most hard-drug users have previous experience with cannabis is not proof that cannabis physically or pharmacologically made them more likely to try a harder drug. Perhaps discovering that the dangers of cannabis were greatly exaggerated by well-meaning drug educators contributed to a conclusion that the dangers reported with harder drugs are also exaggerated. In this case, it would not be cannabis but misinformation about cannabis that "caused" people to progress to harder drugs. Receiving fear-based misinformation about cannabis could be seen as the "gateway" to further rebellion. Furthermore, cannabis is only one leg on the triad; alcohol and tobacco also usually precede progression to harder drug use. Why does cannabis receive the entire blame? The overemphasis of cannabis's role is simply because cannabis is an "illicit drug," which is an arbitrary distinction created by law, not science.

A close look at the gateway theory of progression from softer to harder drugs has never met the rigid scientific criteria used to prove cause and effect. Careful studies of all the factors influencing drug use reveal that, although there is a moderate relationship between early teen cannabis use and later abuse of harder drugs, this association fades when adjustments are made to account for a variety of stressors, such as employment status. In other words, there are many gateways into addiction to hard drugs. To the extent that cannabis use is one of them, it may just be that cannabis is used for the same underlying reasons harder drugs are used later in life. The far, far higher rate of cannabis use compared with harder drugs suggests that the gateway theory has been used more to scare cannabis users than to explain the science of harder drug use. The gateway theory's focus on cannabis as the cause of later drug problems stigmatizes cannabis. Perhaps the gateway theory makes sense to many people, but it does not hold up under the rigorous demands of scientific logic.

As liberal as the Cannabis Culture seems to be about drug use, it fears that any acknowledgment of cannabis's addictive potential would seriously stigmatize their drug of choice. No one wants to be addicted because it is seen as a dark mark against their character. Cannabis Culture is especially reluctant to acknowledge that medical use of cannabis is just as likely as recreational use to lead to addiction. Our brain's cannabinoid receptors and reward system do not care if THC is taken for recreational or medical reasons. Proper use of any medication must include awareness of its potential side effects. When addiction is known to be a potential side effect, protection of the medicine's benefits depends on skillfully managing that addictive potential. The medical community is actually more advanced in its view that cannabis addiction is a disease, not a character flaw, although some doctors do unfortunately still permit their personal biases to contaminate their judgment. Addiction results from a drug's ability to disorder the brain. A person's character ought to be judged more by how they respond to having developed addiction than by the fact that addiction has happened to them.

Conclusion

Having trained in the medical field, I approach addiction as non-judgmentally as I possibly can. THC has less to do with the cause of cannabis addiction than how a person's brain reacts to it. For largely genetic reasons, some people's brains downregulate cannabinoid receptors more quickly, upregulate them more slowly, and dump more dopamine into their reward system in reaction to THC than other brains do. In fact, genetic differences in the number of cannabinoid receptors can be as large as 20 percent. People simply possess different levels of susceptibility to addiction. If the Cannabis Culture and the cannabis industry understood that cannabis addiction is a brain disorder, they would work to protect legalization by acknowledging the risks of use and teaching people how to know their brain's limits. As long as we continue to stigmatize addiction the way Christopher's coach did, rather than treat it as a medical condition requiring understanding and deserving treatment, we will never make the progress needed to help people "Know Your Limits."

12 ADOLESCENTS AND CANNABIS

Stefan's well-educated parents emigrated from the Balkans when Stefan was an infant to escape the violence tearing through their country. He grew up feeling different from his friends. His parents spoke with an accent, didn't automatically understand American customs, and insisted on taking Stefan back to Croatia during summer breaks to visit family after the violence ended. He didn't fit into his parents' homeland or his own new home. He felt fundamentally different from his parents and yet deeply bound to them. Betwixt and between, he was confused by having to face the world on his own.

By middle school, Stefan had already found his way to cannabis. Never a heavy user, he nevertheless adopted a sense of identity from hanging out with fellow pot smokers. Together, they formed an informal fraternity, each opposing the rest of the world for their own personal reasons. No matter how much his parents tried to keep Stefan close to the family and their values, his open pot use at home emphasized his difference from them. At the same time, his use permitted him to join his friends' vague rebellion against American society's norms. Stefan felt self-contained when he was high, and he didn't have to get stoned very often to be defined by its use. He had found more of a home in Cannabis Culture than anywhere else.

When his parents became alarmed that they could not curb Stefan's cannabis use, they asked me to see him. I found Stefan to be intelligent, superficially charming but difficult to meet on *a deeper level, and not using cannabis to a dangerous degree for his brain. And yet, weed was playing an outsized role in his life for the amount he used. He enjoyed denigrating his parents' "pathetic" efforts to act like normal Americans. He understood American culture far better than his parents did, and he rejected much of its demands. He felt suspended outside every cultural norm, except for the ill-defined freedom he found among his friends in the Cannabis Culture.*

Adolescents must be considered a separate subpopulation in any discussion of the effects of cannabis. While most public debate about the increased risks of cannabis use for adolescents properly focuses on their still-developing brains, more detail would be useful. This chapter digs deeper to answer important questions. What does brain development mean? What areas of the brain are still developing during adolescence? What new mental abilities develop as the brain matures? What psychological tasks need to be completed to move from childhood to early adulthood? How does cannabis use alter completion of these tasks during adolescence?

Parents need to understand the answers to these questions, as do teachers and policy makers. Perhaps most importantly, adolescents themselves need this information. The legacy of Reagan's "Just Say No" campaign remains with us. Such simplistic approaches underestimate the natural curiosity and penetrating intelligence of children and teens. Young people have a right to be given all the information they need to make sense of their experience and their world. Full access to such information is crucial to their ability to make healthy choices for themselves. The authoritarian "Just Say No" message is neither a positive step toward developing independent thought nor particularly effective as a prevention strategy. Adolescents deserve real information, and adults need to provide sophisticated, science-based reasons that cannabis use is riskier for youth than for adults.

So, what should parents tell their children about cannabis, and when? What are parents to do when their child experiments with cannabis or becomes devoted to pot? The frustration and pain of watching a teenager fall into the gravitational orbit of Cannabis Culture can be intense. Some parents avoid these uncomfortable feelings by keeping their heads in the sand, finding excuses and reasons to dismiss clear evidence that addiction is driving a wedge between themselves and their child. Others strive to control their child's behavior with increasingly severe punishments, but they soon find that punitive strategies borrowed from the War on Drugs are no more effective within the family than they were for the country as a whole. In their efforts to regain control, parents can become irritable and unreasonable without knowing it as they lose perspective in the midst of their shame, guilt, and impotent fury. This cycle often drives the wedge deeper.

This chapter explores (1) the process of brain development during adolescence, (2) the new cognitive abilities that emerge as the brain develops, (3) the high rate and speed of addiction to cannabis among adolescents, (4) changes in adolescent brain structure caused by regular cannabis use, (5) the cognitive impact of cannabis in adolescents, (6) cannabis's impact on adolescent psychological development, (7) practical impacts on education, career, and general welfare, (8) support for parents with an adolescent addicted to cannabis, and (9) a few notes on the potential impacts of prenatal exposure to cannabis.

Adolescent Brain Development

Puberty initiates a surge of development in both the gray and white matter of the brain. Nerve cell bodies making up gray matter experience a massive growth in the number of synapses, while the long axons making up white matter become insulated to safeguard and speed transmission of signals between parts of the brain. The flourishing growth of synaptic connections can best be visualized as similar to the wild springtime growth of new branches in trees and bushes. Almost overnight, new twigs appear and randomly cross over each other every which way as the plant seeks out every available ray of sunlight. Skilled gardeners know how to improve the health of their plants by pruning away new growth that interferes with established limbs or wastes the plant's energy by growing toward shaded areas. New growth offers new opportunities, and pruning increases the plant's health by strengthening only the most useful new branches.

A well-balanced ECS is intimately involved in regulating the growth and pruning of synapses in the adolescent brain. Synapses occur where the branching end of axons meet the dendrites extending from nerve cell bodies. The onset of puberty causes an increase in axon branching and dendrite growth, resulting in new synaptic connections. Our ECS organizes this growth by guiding construction of the cell's internal scaffolding, which is composed of tiny tubules that stabilize the structure of axons and dendrites. When activated by anandamide and 2-AG, cannabinoid receptors on the tubules respond by lengthening the scaffolding to push dendrites out to connect with axons from upstream neurons. The process is reversed when synapses are pruned by dismantling the scaffolding.

Axons can be thought of as wires. They pass minute electrical impulses from neuron cell bodies to synapses on distant neurons. These wires need to be insulated to work properly, just as the electric wires in your home need to be insulated. The insulation wrapped around axons is a fatty substance called myelin. Myelin enables electric impulses to travel down axons faster and more reliably. Myelin's insulation of axons is jump-started by puberty, along with growth in the number of synapses. Once again, the ECS is intimately involved, as anandamide and

2-AG guide the process of myelination. Throughout our lives, endocannabinoids and their receptors work to repair and maintain myelin insulation around axons. Too much cannabinoid activation by THC interferes with proper myelin health. Without good myelination, connections between neurons are impaired.

The "gardener" for the new synapses in a teen's brain is experience and learning. Synapses activated by experience and learning are strengthened, while those not activated will wither. Adolescent brain development is thus a process of both rapid synaptic expansion and gradual pruning. Eventually, a single neuron can receive signals from as many as 10,000 other neurons, while its own axon reaches out to connect with up to 10,000 other neurons. The resulting complexity may be mind-numbing to conceptualize, but it is literally mind-vitalizing and expanding for the adolescent.

The pruning necessary for maturation does not happen simultaneously throughout the brain. MRIs of the outer cortex layer of the brain show that maturation begins at the back of the brain and advances forward. The last areas to mature are the frontal lobes. Full maturation is generally considered complete by age 25; it is no coincidence that this is the age when car rental companies no longer levy a surcharge.

New Cognitive Abilities with Brain Maturation

Neanderthals coexisted and even bred with modern *Homo sapiens*, until their extinction 40,000 years ago. When I examine reconstructions of Neanderthal faces, my attention focuses on their backward-sloping foreheads. This skull configuration offers a window into understanding the critical brain development that separates modern humans from earlier versions. Our forehead has been pushed out by the most recent evolutionary development in the mammalian brain: our expanded frontal lobes. Without the development of frontal lobes, the modern mind would not exist.

As our frontal lobes mature, our highest cognitive functions spring to life to increase our intellectual capacity and transform the regulation of emotion. Generally grouped together under the term "executive functions," these new cognitive abilities become progressively more available with postpubertal brain maturation. One way to conceptualize the role executive functions play is to look at what happens when they are lost. During the mid-twentieth century, the lack of effective psychiatric treatment for severe mental disorders led to the advent of psychosurgical procedures, such as frontal lobotomies that disconnected the frontal lobes from the rest of the brain. Frontal lobotomies eliminate our executive functioning skills, resulting in what physicians described as "surgically induced childhood." Ken Kesey's *One Flew Over the Cuckoo's Nest* graphically dramatized lobotomies. I did a portion of my psychiatric training in the same locked unit where Kesey worked when he wrote *Cuckoo's Nest*. It was there that I met the only lobotomized patient I have ever encountered. A genial, pliable man, he had little impulse control and got into trouble for attacking another patient who greeted him one morning with the raised fist of solidarity popular at the time. Without the executive function of his frontal lobe, my patient could not distinguish this friendly greeting from a threatening gesture. I explained how a raised fist has different meanings in different contexts, but he was never able to grasp this concept. Like a young child, he was unable to shift his perspective on the basis of sophisticated social cues. After his lobotomy, he lost the ability to think abstractly and was consigned to a very concrete interpretation of the world.

Executive functions include the ability to interpret events within the context they occur and to focus on high-priority stimuli while ignoring distractions. Executive functions give us better impulse control and decision-making skills. The development of more abstract thinking improves prioritizing, planning, sequencing, and judgment. Self-awareness deepens when we are able to see ourselves in the broader context of our family and the community as a whole. Greater mental flexibility is achieved when contradictory thoughts and feelings can be entertained, perspective can be shifted with new information, and emotional regulation is aided by cognitive understanding. Emotional reactivity begins to be tempered when it occurs within the context of a more abstract understanding that is provided by maturing frontal lobes. When balance between the two is achieved, a mature personality capable of both intellectual understanding and emotional intelligence is ready to step into the world of adulthood. Exactly how neural activity in the frontal lobes generates these executive functions remains a mystery, but no more of a mystery than how neural activity in the occipital lobe cortex at the back of the brain generates vision. Nevertheless, we are certain that healthy, mature gray matter in the frontal lobes and occipital cortex is necessary for executive functions and vision to exist.

With the proper growth and pruning of synapses in the frontal lobes, and with the proper myelin insulation of axons, adolescents gain access to a more complex view of themselves and the world. In addition, with strengthened connection between the frontal lobe and the amygdala and hippocampus, the new executive functions can interact with emotions and memory, respectively. Adolescents gain the ability to regulate impulses, urges, and emotions.

As Stefan began puberty, his understanding of the disparities between his experience and world view and that of his parents became more complex and acute. His ill-defined childhood feeling of being different only deepened and became more intense and discomforting. Neural

maturation thrust him into new and more complex awareness. Without anyone understanding the uniqueness of
his experience, he felt more fundamentally isolated than
ever. The psychological challenges that served as a road-
block to adulthood began to seem insurmountable.

Increased Risk of Addiction for Adolescents

It would be incorrect to imply that the increased rate
and speed of addiction to cannabis during adolescence is
disproportionately greater than for other drugs, such as
tobacco, alcohol, opiates, and stimulants. For a variety
of physical and emotional reasons, adolescents simply
become addicted to drugs far more rapidly and at
a greater rate than adults. Addiction to the triad of tobacco,
alcohol, and cannabis looms largest for adolescents primarily because of their greater availability. The *average*
age of cannabis use onset ranges from a low of 13.5 years
among Native Americans to a high of 16.8 years among
Asian Americans, with other racial groups falling in
between. As this is the average age of onset, many young-
sters begin using much earlier.

   Figure 12.1 illustrates the increased risk of adolescents
becoming dependent on cannabis. Each bar represents the
percentage dependent at a given age for individuals who
began use 2 years earlier. For example, 17.4 percent of
individuals who began cannabis use at age 11 meet the
criteria for a diagnosis of CUD (i.e. dependence/addiction)
by 13 years of age. Among those who begin at 13 years,
16.4 percent are dependent by age 15. As the age of onset
increases, the graph shows a gradual decrease in the
percentage who become addicted within 2 years. Only
3 percent of those who wait until 20 develop dependence
by age 22. The earlier adolescents begin using cannabis, the
more likely they are to quickly become addicted. As with

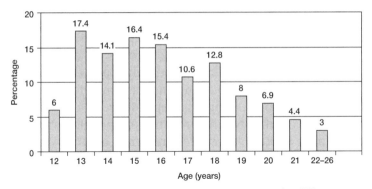

Figure 12.1 Rate of cannabis dependence in past year for different ages of onset of use.

all drugs, the onset of cannabis use before impulse control is fully matured increases the risk of addiction.

When adolescent users are followed beyond 2 years, the percentage who become dependent continues to rise over time. By 18 years old, 28 percent of those who started use at 13 have become addicted, 34 percent by 21, and a full 43 percent by age 30. These are called lifetime dependence rates, meaning that a person has been addicted at some point during their lifetime. When adolescents delay the onset of use, even for a few years, lifetime rates are much lower. For example, those who start using at 15 have a 25 percent lifetime rate of addiction by 30, but those who begin at age 19 have only a 15 percent lifetime dependence rate by age 30.

Lifetime rates are often used to emphasize the seriousness of drug addiction. As addiction specialists like to say, "If left untreated, addiction is a disease that ends in insanity or death." This belief passes as conventional wisdom among many mental health professionals who treat the most serious cases of alcohol, opiate, or methamphetamine addiction. It is unfortunately true that professionals have watched millions of lives spiral toward inevitable destruction when addicts are unable to abstain from alcohol and hard drugs. But the data simply do not support this dire fate for most people who experience a period of cannabis dependence. Only 15 percent of adolescents who begin cannabis use at 13 and only 9 percent of those who begin at 15 are addicted during the year before turning 30. In other words, cannabis dependence is not usually a lifelong condition. The majority of people who use frequently enough to cause problems only do so for a discrete period of their lives. For most people, including the majority who develop dependence, cannabis misuse is a phase. Use that falls short of addiction also tends to be a phase. Data show that 82 percent of people who use cannabis at least ten times stop by age 34, the majority reporting that they merely lost interest in the drug.

A 15 percent rate of addiction at age 30 for those who started using at 13 is clearly not a good thing. It's very likely that the course of life for these 15 percent has been significantly and negatively impacted by cannabis. Even those who were cannabis dependent in their early adolescence and then stopped using or cut back enough to no longer satisfy criteria for CUD could be suffering limited career opportunities because of critical disruptions to their education.

Altered Brain Structure with Regular Cannabis Use

Adolescents who use cannabis heavily affect the development of both gray and white matter in their brains. The largest area of gray matter is the complexly folded cortex that covers the surface of the brain; a tenth of an inch thick and containing roughly 25 billion neuron cell bodies, the cortex would be the size of a newspaper's front page if flattened out. Other collections of gray matter, such as the amygdala, hippocampus, basal ganglia, reward center, and hypothalamus, exist partially or completely beneath the surface cortex. What people generally think of as "nerves" are tracts of axons running together, for example, from the spinal cord out to different muscles, passing electrical impulses at up to 275 miles (442 km) per hour. There are also tracts of axons within the brain, connecting different areas of gray matter. The largest nerve tract within the brain connects and coordinates the left and right hemispheres. Saddled with the clumsy name, "corpus callosum," this massive tract contains over 200 million axons running in both directions like a superhighway.

Regular cannabis use leads to a 20 percent reduction in available cannabinoid receptors in the cortex, although the majority of this reduction is reversed within several days of abstinence. However, this research was conducted with adult users, leaving us uncertain whether adolescents are more or less affected, and whether receptor downregulation is as quickly reversed with abstinence.

Changes in the volume of gray matter are seen throughout the brains of cannabis users. One of the most consistent findings reveals a smaller hippocampal volume in cannabis users relative to non-users – 12 percent smaller on average. A study of London cab drivers nicely illustrated that the hippocampus is the basic neural machinery for memory. The longer any individual drove through the maze of streets in this ancient city, memorizing each alley and shortcut, the larger their hippocampus grew. But animal studies show that THC reduces the number of synapses in the hippocampus by 44 percent and shortens the length of dendrites, both of which would contribute to smaller volume and decreased memory. It should be noted that individuals who used cannabis with higher amounts of CBD had smaller reductions in hippocampal volume, demonstrating the neuroprotective nature of CBD. The amygdala, the biological center for emotion, appetite, and novelty, is also reduced in volume by 7 percent in cannabis users, and changes in the shape of the reward center occur with regular use.

The volume of gray matter in the surface cortex gradually declines from the onset of puberty through early adulthood (age 25) as a result of pruning. When cannabis is used before age 16, the frontal cortex is thicker than normal, probably due to a reduction in pruning. More synapses remain, whether they are activated by experience or not. However, in the case of a thicker frontal cortex, bigger is not necessarily better. Brains need to be pruned every bit as much as trees and bushes do to be healthy. With an onset of cannabis use after age 16, the frontal cortex is thinner than normal. This discrepancy between onset of use before and after age 16 illustrates the existence of critical periods during brain development. Cannabis use during a critical period, when changes in brain structure are happening most rapidly and basic structural patterns are first being created, can be far more consequential than use during later periods. This is no different from how problems with the foundation of a house weaken the entire structure built upon it.

White matter is also affected by cannabis use, although the consequences for our brain health are harder to outline. In addition to conducting electric impulses from nerve cell bodies to synapses, axon microtubules also transport water and important molecular cargo to these synapses. Typical neurotransmitters, such as serotonin and dopamine, are synthesized in nerve cell bodies and need to be carried down the full length of axons to where they are released at synapses. Highly sophisticated imaging technology can analyze the flow of water through axons, which normally occurs exclusively in one direction, from cell bodies to synapses. THC disrupts the structure of microtubules by creating unneeded branching. When the microtubule scaffolding is disrupted, the integrity and efficiency of axons is damaged and the transmission of electrical impulses is impaired. Water no longer carries its molecular cargo as efficiently. This disruption is especially apparent in the portion of the corpus callosum that is made up of axons connecting the frontal lobes on either side of the brain. The damage was observed to occur in 16–18-year-olds who previously used little cannabis but became regular users during these 3 years.

In one illuminating study, the clever modification of an Etch A Sketch revealed one consequence of cannabis-induced damage to axons in the corpus callosum. When asked to use the two knobs to move a cursor through a narrow maze, regular cannabis users are slower and have poorer coordination between their two hands. These impairments are the result of less information passing between the two hemispheres, each of which controls only one hand. Clear communication between the left and right sides of the brain is necessary for good physical coordination. We can only wonder how impaired integration of high-order executive functions between the two hemispheres may contribute to cognitive difficulties.

Changes in the brain's structure lead to changes in its function, and changes in brain function impact the mind. None of the changes in gray and white matter outlined above would be significant unless changes in mental function also occur. We can now turn to the cognitive changes that result from THC's impact on the brain.

Cognitive Impact of Cannabis in Adolescence

The impact of cannabis use has been studied less thoroughly in adolescents than in adults. As a result, many findings have been documented only in adults, leaving us to presume they also occur in adolescents. Such presumptions are likely to be correct but lack real scientific rigor. This section looks at data gathered from adolescent-only studies and leaves the bulk of what has been discovered in adults for Chapter 13.

Neurocognitive testing reveals a range of impairments in adolescents who use cannabis regularly, with significantly poorer results found among early-onset users (before age 16). Two tests, the Wisconsin Card Sort and the Stroop test, illustrate the difficulties created by cannabis particularly well. In the Wisconsin Card Sort, participants are asked to match cards without knowing the rule for the match. Each card has colorful symbols in varying numbers (e.g. three yellow triangles, one blue circle, four red stars). Three obvious ways of classifying the cards are apparent (by color, shape, or number), but only one is deemed correct. With each effort to match the cards, participants are only told if they are correct or not. The classification rule changes every so often, and the subject is only alerted to the change when the previous rule no longer yields the correct answer. The way of sorting that was once correct is suddenly wrong. How long does it take the participant to discover the new sorting strategy, and how long do they keep trying to make the old strategy work? The Wisconsin Card Sort is an excellent measure of mental flexibility. The earlier an adolescent has started using cannabis, the less mental flexibility they possess and the lower their score on the test.

The Stroop test is even more devilish. After being sure the subject is not color blind, they are presented a list of color names (e.g. red, blue) that are printed in a color that does not match (e.g. the word red printed in blue ink). They are asked to ignore the word and name the color of ink. This is an excellent measure of one's ability to concentrate on one thing while filtering out and ignoring distractions. As with the Wisconsin Card Sort, early-onset cannabis users receive lower scores than late-onset users, and both do more poorly than non-users. The Stroop test documents both slower processing speed and an increase in incorrect responses. These lower scores are the result of a decreased ability to maintain divided attention and suppress intrusive distractions, called interferences. Many a stoned conversation has veered hilariously from one topic to another without a coherent through line as random thoughts "intrude" partway through a sentence.

While additional ways of measuring executive functions exist and have been used to demonstrate the impairments caused by cannabis, I will focus on the Go/No-Go protocol measure of impulsivity, which is an inability to suppress undesirable responses. One example of the Go/No-Go test asks subjects to push a button as quickly as possible when any letter appears on a computer screen except an "X." When an "X" appears, they are not to push the button. Adolescent cannabis users perform as accurately as nonusers, with no higher a rate of impulsive responses. However, brain imaging reveals that larger areas of the cortex are active during this task in cannabis users. Researchers believe cannabis users have increased difficulty with this task and compensate by recruiting a larger area of the brain to avoid impulsively committing incorrect responses. Adults with documented damage to their white matter from cannabis use show a measurable increase in impulsivity in the Go/No-Go test, proving that impulsivity is a consequence of cannabis use. At an older age, adults appear to lack the ability to activate a larger portion of the cortex to compensate for their impairment as well as adolescents.

Perhaps the best-known study of the impact cannabis has on adolescents' cognitive ability is known as the Dunedin study, named after the town in New Zealand where over 1,000 people born in the early 1970s were followed for the next 35 years. The study found as much as an 8-point decline in IQ in individuals between age 13 and 35 when regular cannabis use began in their early teens and continued throughout the study. IQ measurement is a composite of numerous neurocognitive tests, including many that measure executive function. The decline in IQ found in early-onset, ongoing cannabis users resulted from impairment in memory and executive function tests, like the Wisconsin Card Sort and the Stroop test.

Unfortunately, the Dunedin study has been misinterpreted by many who wish to emphasize the risks of using cannabis. While the study documented cognitive impairments in early-onset users, it also clearly showed that regular cannabis use starting after late adolescence does *not* result in lower IQ scores. The only permanent cognitive deficits Dunedin proved result from early-onset use.

This is bad news for early adolescents who become devoted to cannabis. Further bad news is that executive function impairment lingers longer after stopping use for adolescent users than for adults. Executive functions remain below normal for a month after adolescents stop use when compared with non-users of the same age, while adults have reversed the impairment after about a week. Even more bad news: sensitive studies now show measurable executive function deficits with as little as once-weekly use.

Cannabis and Adolescent Psychological Development

I do not envy American youth today, growing up in fear of climate change, embroiled in racial and gender identity issues, in a time of gross economic disparity and insecurity, buffeted by a global pandemic of uncertain duration and educational disruption, and with contradictory role models offered by political leaders, Obama/Biden and Trump. In the midst of this disorienting national and global uncertainty, waves of preteens continue to be thrust into adolescence, their bodies resculpted and minds shaken and turbocharged by puberty. These changes push them into new challenges, willingly or not. The basic psychological developmental tasks of adolescence remain what they have always been despite the new circumstances in which these tasks must be undertaken. As always, satisfactory completion of these interlocking developmental tasks is necessary in order to launch successfully into adulthood.

During the decade following the onset of puberty, each person must develop in the following four broad psychological areas:

- Autonomy and separation.
- Identity and values.
- Peer group attachment.
- Transcendence.

Adolescents need to develop a sense of autonomy that is independent from their parents. Even when they choose to follow in their parents' footsteps, maturation requires that each adolescent choose this life course for their own internal reasons. A simplistic way to declare separation from one's parents is to become the opposite, but this stance still keeps parents at the center of your outwardly rebellious identity. Instead, a more mature and authentic identity needs to be forged out of one's own freely chosen values. But what are one's own values? This question is partially answered by choices in peer relationships. Attaching to a peer group substantially adds to an adolescent's sense of autonomy, easing the process of separating from the family identity. In the best circumstances, affiliation with a peer group does not supplant connection to parents but rather opens one's horizons to include attachment to a much wider world. The conflicting attachment to family and peers is eased by parents who foster their child's autonomy. Ultimately, most adolescents are able to develop their own sense of identity beyond parental control, without disconnecting from the family ties that can keep them firmly grounded while allowing them to develop psychologically. Adolescence can be tumultuous, but turmoil is not necessary for full psychological development to occur.

In addition to establishing autonomy from parents, developing one's identity with a clear sense of values, and forging intimate attachments to peers outside the family, most adolescents also have a need for transcendence. Bereft of the simplistic, magical perspective of childhood and far from the competence and power of adulthood, adolescents long to transcend their position in the off-stage wings of life. With growing awareness of the hypocrisy and pretense among adults that comes with increasingly abstract thinking, they long to create a more perfect world to live in. Suddenly unsure of life's meaning and no longer comforted by childish beliefs in Santa Claus or religious ideas they previously accepted without question, all the cards in the deck they played with as children are thrown into the air. Adolescence is a way station rife with uncertainty and suffused with the singular purpose of maturing beyond one's simplistic childhood identity. A longing to transcend one's present circumstances leads many adolescents to have a natural curiosity about anything that fosters new horizons of consciousness.

Drugs offer an easy vehicle for transcendence. While tobacco offers symbolic relief from mere adolescence and alcohol offers the relief of gaiety and being comfortably numb, cannabis is something altogether different. Cannabis offers a sense of expanded consciousness, and Cannabis Culture offers an exciting haven.

The moment a teen decides to smoke their first joint, they experience stepping unequivocally out of their childhood, beyond the wishes and confines of their parents and traditional society, and into a new peer group that unconditionally accepts their belonging. They have taken on a new identity: risk-taker, explorer, outlaw, adventurer, deep thinker. It's easy for some adolescents to be enthralled with cannabis when it feels simultaneously joyful, fascinating, and stress relieving, and offers a new community, ego-transcending spirituality, and a shortcut to meeting the challenges of psychological development. The act of using cannabis feels like a personal, autonomous decision that breaks from parental expectations. It instantly supplies a new facet to one's identity. Cannabis Culture supports a whole new perspective on the world with its own set of values. Acceptance into a new peer group, with its own secrets and language, confirms the transition to a new identity. Cannabis provides a sense of transcendence on many levels: childhood has been transcended with a leap into adult pleasures, old norms are transcended, and for many, the sense of teenage disconnection and isolation is transcended, as though the limiting boundaries of subjective experience itself have been shed. Mystical interconnectedness seems possible. All this is accomplished without doing the hard, internal, psychological work needed to weather the pressures encountered in adulthood and establish deeply rooted autonomy, separation, identity, values, and intimate affiliation with healthy peers. I am speaking of those adolescents who move from experimental use to committed, devoted cannabis use. Only a minority of adolescents who ever use cannabis travel this route, but it is an important minority. As noted previously, over 16 percent of adolescents who begin using cannabis by age 13 show signs of addiction within the next 2 years, and 15 percent of that group are still addicted at age 30. These are the youth most likely to have their psychological development derailed by regular cannabis use.

Cannabis provides an imitation of maturation, but the roots are too shallow to survive. While cannabis can reveal a universe of new possibilities, it does not help an adolescent *realize* any of these possibilities. For adolescents who lack the life experience useful for resisting the allure of such temptations, and especially for those who are genetically prone toward addiction, cannabis may seem like the key that unlocks their way into a different world. They see the finger pointing the way and then suck it with delight rather than follow the direction it points.

Stefan was dancing at the edge of a risky precipice. He did not use enough cannabis to permanently alter his brain, but he permitted it to play too big a role in his psychological development to be safe. His need to resolve the conundrum of being caught between two worlds was interrupted by a detour to nowhere offered by cannabis's seductive fantasies of maturity. Stefan ran the risk of finding himself still caught in adolescence when most of his peers had moved on to adult perspectives. He needed guidance but had closed himself off from his "old world" parents. He needed a good therapist who could challenge his judgment and serve as a compass toward a realistic future. And he needed a therapist to keep tabs on his cannabis use and teach him how to keep it from getting out of control.

Practical Impacts of Cannabis on Education, Career, and General Welfare

Just as there are critical periods in brain development, adolescence is a critical period in psychological development that affects the overall trajectory of our adult life. When youth become overinvolved with cannabis use for a few years, it can have a profound enough impact on their academic performance to alter prospects for subsequent education, training, and employment. The question is no longer whether an adolescent has become addicted to cannabis, but rather whether their being in thrall to it has interrupted their ability to earn the tickets needed to launch into an economically and socially successful adulthood. Once established in a stable job and intimate partnership, adults can often coast for a few years of over-involvement with cannabis without becoming completely derailed. When their use of cannabis stops, they have a solid enough foundation to fall back on. In contrast, if adolescents get lost in cannabis use, they will lack this fundamental foundation of education and skills when their interest in cannabis wanes. It will be too late to go back to high school, and they will be old enough that they need to support themselves financially however they can as an untrained worker.

This bleak outlook is not offered as a fear tactic; it stems from data. While I have known high-school students who used cannabis regularly and went on to prestigious universities and successful careers, they have beaten the odds and defied the statistics. Adolescents who use cannabis 100 times are almost six times more likely to drop out of school. It's not hard to use cannabis 100 times – just once a week for 2 years, twice a week for 1 year, or once or twice a day for the summer vacation. Non-users are over three times more likely to attend college. An interesting natural experiment shines a light on these statistics. When Maastricht, a university town in the Netherlands, prevented foreign students from purchasing cannabis at local "coffee shops" for 4 months, their grades and pass rates went up with no greater study time. This boost in academic achievement was lost after the ban on sales was lifted.

Among New Zealanders in the Dunedin study with high cannabis use between ages 14 and 21, a wide range of negative outcomes occurred by age 25. The income of those who used cannabis 400 times or more was 76 percent that of non-users. Welfare dependence was 3.6 times higher. Unemployment was 2.6 times higher. Self-reported relationship and overall life satisfaction were lower. Cause and effect are not clear with these statistics, and it can be argued that many people with a less-than-satisfying life might welcome the balm that cannabis offers. A study in the Boston area contributed to the growing body of knowledge on the adverse consequences suffered by heavy cannabis users between ages 30 and 55. While the levels of education and income in families of origin were similar for heavy users and non-users, users had significantly lower levels of educational achievement and income. By self-report, 90 percent felt that cannabis had a "negative effect" on their cognition and memory, 79 percent on career, 70 percent on social life, 81 percent on physical health, and 60 percent on mental health. The earlier the onset of use, the more likely it is that an individual will become a long-term user with a long-term impact on quality of life.

Support for Parents with a Child Addicted to Cannabis

Parents can have a variety of reactions to learning that their child is addicted to cannabis. Some ignore or rationalize it. Some worry, nag, plead, or beg their child to quit. Some are horribly alarmed, clamp down, yell, monitor, and try to control their child with demands and punishments. But almost all parents are embarrassed and keep the problem as quiet as possible. Few parents have extensive knowledge about cannabis, although many have experienced it themselves. Whether they should share their own experience with cannabis is often a haunting question. In the end, perhaps the most difficult thing for parents to accept is that their child is an independent being with a separate mind that cannot be coerced. While parents may be able to reward or force their child's behavior to comply with their wishes, they are ultimately powerless to control a child's mind.

The most powerful resource for parents with an addicted child is Al-Anon, an offshoot of Alcoholics Anonymous in which family members and friends of loved ones with an alcohol or drug problem gather for mutual support. Being among peers who are facing the same problem and who have tried the same unsuccessful solutions breaks the isolation and dissolves the embarrassment many parents feel. Al-Anon embodies the hard-won wisdom that we only add fuel to the fire when our own exasperation results in futile and unreasonable behavior. For example, making exaggerated, empty threats only diminishes whatever authority you have left with your child, and yet, it is hard not to threaten dire consequences out of frustration and an impending sense of impotence. Al-Anon provides a path capable of keeping reactions to an addicted child reasonable and loving.

The Al-Anon program focuses on discerning what can and cannot be controlled. It proposes accepting powerlessness over what is impossible to control as the starting point for responding to another's addiction. The program also emphasizes being open to help from other sources, including faith in a "higher power" of your own definition. Al-Anon does not, however, offer concrete advice or direction. For more pragmatic matters such as formal medical/psychological evaluations and treatment resources, it is best to meet with a professional trained in addiction medicine. The American Society of Addiction Medicine and reputable local treatment centers can provide recommendations for professionals with specialized training. It is difficult to be an informed consumer of mental health or substance abuse services, especially during a family crisis. The best referrals are often found through the network of parents at Al-Anon meetings, particularly at meetings with a parental focus.

Prenatal Exposure to Cannabis

We all begin life as a single cell. We are the egg that ripened in our mother's ovary plus the chromosomes that were delivered in the sperm lucky enough to have fertilized the egg. Soon, the fertilized egg splits into two cells, then each splits into two more. As cells grow and divide again and again, each new cell carries precisely the same genes as all the others. Instead of simply becoming a larger and larger ball of identical cells, some cells begin to differentiate. After 4 weeks have passed, a groove appears on the embryo's surface, deepens, folds over itself, and becomes a tube. This tube eventually becomes the spinal cord, and one end of that tube becomes our brain. As miraculous as this seems, it is so ingrained in the nature of early embryonic cells that the same process takes place in every fish, frog, snake, bird, and mammal. Once the basic neural structure is created, individual nerve cells continue to divide, migrate, and extend their axons out to connect with each other. By age 3, the human brain is already 85 percent the size it will be in adulthood. This first period of rapid brain development ends, and further mental growth depends largely on learning and the accumulation of experience until a second period of structural change begins at puberty.

Only a few scientists have investigated the effect of cannabis exposure on fetal brain development. I think of fetal exposure to cannabis as "second-hand cannabis," like the second-hand smoke exposure cigarettes create for people sitting near a smoker. In 2012, average cannabis use during the three trimesters of pregnancy was reported to be 9 percent, 5 percent, and 2.4 percent, respectively. Unfortunately, the first trimester is a critical period for laying down the basic foundation of our nervous system. Half of women using cannabis during pregnancy do so to relieve nausea and vomiting, which is worst during the first trimester. Women who believe cannabis is a safe treatment for morning sickness likely don't know that THC concentrations in the fetus are approximately one-third of what is measured in the mother's blood. A Scottish study found THC in the meconium (an infant's first intestinal discharge) of over 13 percent of newborns. As many as 28 percent of young, urban, disadvantaged women use cannabis during pregnancy. Prenatal exposure to cannabis is widespread, and fortunately, no major birth defects are known to result from prenatal exposure to cannabis.

Maternal cannabis use is important because fetal nerve cell migration, axonal wiring, and development of synapses are all guided by our ECS. Anandamide and 2-AG levels are five times higher in fetal brains than in those of adults, and they activate CB1 receptors at the leading edge of axonal growth to build the scaffolding that directs neurons to their proper destination. Introducing THC at this critical period of fetal brain development causes branching in this scaffolding, decreasing axonal integrity.

Long-term studies, beginning with an assessment of cannabis use during pregnancy and continuing for the first two decades of a child's life, are difficult, expensive, and require persistent dedication throughout a researcher's career. Such studies are therefore rare. Only three have been conducted for long enough to provide data, but they differed so greatly in their methodology and populations studied that none of their results have been independently validated. Nevertheless, these studies clearly show that there are a variety of measurable cognitive deficits throughout childhood, adolescence, and early adulthood in individuals exposed to second-hand cannabis while still in their mother's womb.

Deficits include impaired mental development at 9 months, impaired abstract reasoning and short-term memory at 3 years, impaired memory and verbal development at 4 years, and impaired attention and impulse control with hyperactivity at 6 years. When higher cognitive abilities begin to mature in the child and can be more reliably tested, documented adverse consequences of prenatal cannabis exposure include increased hyperactivity, impulsivity, and inattention at 10 years, and impaired executive function and problem solving at 9–12 years. Adverse consequences in adolescence include impaired problem solving and analytic skills that require sustained attention, observed in 13–16-year-olds. From ages 18 to 22, fMRIs performed during working memory and executive function tasks reveal significantly less activity in the frontal lobes and compensatory increased activity in multiple other areas of the cortex.

These results clearly reveal a pattern of difficulties with attention and executive functions throughout childhood and adolescence. Only future research will establish the full extent of the problems caused by prenatal cannabis exposure. Recently released data from an ongoing landmark study of nearly 12,000 children across the USA (the Adolescent Brain Cognition and Development (ABCD) Study) confirm the findings of the three previous long-term studies of the negative impact of cannabis on the fetal brain. Despite the accumulating evidence, fetuses are still being exposed to higher levels of THC than ever. Will the subtle findings reported by early studies become more obvious in newborns over the next two decades? This prospect led the American College of Obstetrics and Gynecology to recommend that the only prudent course of action is to avoid cannabis use during pregnancy.

Conclusion

One indisputable conclusion to draw from the information presented in this chapter is that public health policies need to emphasize the importance of adolescents and pregnant women avoiding, delaying, or decreasing cannabis use. While the goals of avoid, delay, and decrease are clear, there is no clarity about which public health policies would most effectively reach these goals. The principles that might best guide effective public health policy will be explored in Chapter 15.

13 FURTHER CONSEQUENCES OF USING CANNABIS TOO FREQUENTLY

Robert was a successful medical device sales representative. His work was twofold: he educated surgeons about his company's knee and hip replacement hardware, and entertained them with meals and friendly conversation. The more his network of relationships in the medical community grew, the easier his job became. He worked from home half the time and found it easy to use cannabis when his disapproving wife was at work and his kids were in school. He had enjoyed the buzz cannabis gave him since he started using it in college.

Robert came to see me at his wife's insistence after she caught him smoking a joint in the attic one Saturday morning. He said he was up there because he didn't want the children to smell it. His wife was furious because she was about to bring their daughter up to the attic to look for some old pictures. When she called to schedule her husband's appointment, she complained that he was emotionally absent and becoming less careful with hiding his use. When Robert arrived for his session, he started by complaining about his wife's overreaction and then minimized the possibility that cannabis was causing any difficulties in their lives. He claimed that his work was going very well, but eventually revealed almost having lost a big order because he misjudged the risk of adding an extra delivery charge. This upset him because he prided himself on accurately reading customers' needs. I asked if he was willing to listen to some information about the long-term impact of cannabis. He reluctantly said he would listen but admitted that it probably wouldn't change his mind.

I purposefully placed the discussion of the long-term risks of using cannabis beyond the brain's limits toward the end of this book for two reasons. First, many people are reluctant to pay attention to the science of how cannabis works when they believe the information is presented primarily to demonize the drug. Hopefully, I have proven in the previous chapters that I do not oppose all use of cannabis, only its unsafe use. Second, once people have grasped the basic science of cannabis and the brain, they are more open to understanding that any drug with the power to entertain, mystify, and heal is likely to have some negative side effects. This chapter turns a clear eye to what is known about these side effects.

The following consequences of using cannabis too frequently are all documented by multiple high-quality studies of adults who use cannabis regularly, often 20 or more days a month. All research included in this chapter was conducted when participants were not high. Many regular cannabis users report improved memory and problem solving after use, rather than the impairments described below. When this improvement is real, it likely stems from THC's reversal of impairments caused by downregulation of cannabinoid receptors. Testing heavy users after ingesting cannabis shows that THC's strong cannabinoid stimulation can temporarily compensate for this downregulation. There is no doubt that well-chosen cognitive testing of regular cannabis users reveals the following negative consequences when the influence of THC is removed.

Memory

Long-term, regular cannabis users receive lower scores on memory tests than shorter-term users and non-users. These impairments worsen with increased quantity, frequency, and duration of cannabis use. When asked to listen to and then repeat a list of 15 common words, cannabis users underperform. Then, when the list is repeated and recall is measured five more times, the learning curve for users falls below non-user control subjects. After a different list of 15 words is read and the subject's recall is tested, having heard this second list interferes more with regular cannabis users' performance on recall of the initial 15 words than it does with controls. A final recall of the original list after waiting 20 minutes was also worse for users. Between 80 and 90 percent of both short-term (10 years) and long-term (20 years) users acknowledge problems with memory and attention resulting from their use. Adolescents who use cannabis 2–3 days a week for 2–3 years have the same level of memory impairment as adult users with approximately 20 years of use. Research continues to document increasingly subtle memory impairment in early-onset users, even when they use with minimal frequency and smaller amounts of cannabis. Individuals who used cannabis at least once a week before age 16 have been shown to possess reduced verbal learning skills compared with those who began similar use after their 16th birthday.

I need to add that the degree of memory impairment in regular cannabis users is not clinically important. It does not warrant a diagnosis even marginally approaching dementia. However, impairments in regular cannabis users have been shown to have impacts outside the controlled environment of the research laboratory. Distractions and multitasking in the real world are more likely to interfere with memory. Standardized questionnaires given to 21-year-olds with a 3–4-year history of regular cannabis use reveal 20 percent lower scores in measures of everyday memory when compared with non-users. Cognitive failures and forgetfulness can include forgetting the location of familiar objects around the house, failing to recognize acquaintances, or forgetting important events that occurred the previous day. Lapses in remembering to perform future tasks can include forgetting to turn off the lights, attend a meeting, or mail a letter. A 20 percent reduction in working memory can be significant enough to have practical impacts on education, job performance, and relationships.

A healthy hippocampus is necessary for reaching your learning and memory potential. Long-term, regular use of cannabis is known to reduce the number of synapses and the total volume of the hippocampus, with the measurable impacts on memory outlined above.

Executive Function

Our executive functions are essentially what people mean by intelligence. They permit us to mentally manipulate ideas, pause to think before acting, flexibly meet unanticipated challenges, resist temptations, assess risk, and stay focused – all necessary for self-regulation and to achieve goals. Executive functions are not discrete and easily enumerated like the fingers on our hands. Rather, they overlap and are defined by the cognitive tests used to measure them. While neurocognitive testing can measure the existence of these abilities, there is no guarantee they will ever be put to good use. Wisdom is different from intelligence and cannot be measured; just as a quarterback's basic skills can be measured, their savvy during tense game situations is less tangible.

Subtle frontal-lobe deficits can be observed using the Wisconsin Card Sort and the Stroop test, but other basic executive functions are measured by the Digit Symbol Substitution test and the Trail Making test. The Digit Symbol Substitution test provides a set of symbols paired with single-digit numbers; participants are asked to select the proper symbol and copy it next to a list of sample digits. The task is simple, almost like breaking a code. Read the next digit on the list (e.g. 4), look up to the top of the page and see which symbol corresponds to the number 4 (e.g. a plus sign), and then draw a plus next to the number 4 on the list below before moving on to the next number. Subjects are asked to complete as many of these digit/ symbol pairings as possible during the time allotted. When a participant makes more mistakes and copies fewer symbols than average, it can be concluded that their attention, memory, and/or processing speed are below normal. Adults who regularly use cannabis perform below normal for approximately 1 week after becoming abstinent.

The Trail Making test demonstrates subtle deficits in regular cannabis users' ability to sequence and shift focus. Each trial is a simple connect-the-dots exercise. The first trial uses numbers, and the next uses the alphabet. The true test of interest asks the participant to connect dots that alternate between numbers and letters (e.g. 1, A, 2, B, 3, C). When mistakes are made and dots are connected more slowly, it can be concluded that a person's ability to shift between one set (numbers) and another (letters) is impaired and processing speed has decreased. Adults using cannabis regularly require a week of abstinence to regain normal scores, but adolescents require a month. As the results of executive function tests compare average scores for a group of users with average scores for a group of non-using matched controls, they do not predict any given individual's score. There is a bit of overlap, with a few non-users receiving lower scores than a few regular users. But, on average, most regular users lag behind most non-users.

When CB1 receptors in the frontal lobes are suppressed by regular cannabis use, the frontal lobes do not function as well. Subtle deficits in even the most basic executive functions linger for a week in adults and a month in adolescents. When this downregulation of cannabinoid receptors occurs during the neurodevelopmentally critical period of early adolescence, pruning of unused synapses is affected and the impact on cognitive function can be permanent.

Error Awareness

In order to improve performance on any task, we first need to be aware that we have made a mistake. A complex combination of the Go/No-Go and the Stroop tests was designed to measure a person's awareness of having impulsively responded when they should have withheld their response, called the Error Awareness Task. The test presented cards on a computer screen with the names of colors. Sometimes the color names were presented in the same color as the name, and sometimes in a different color. People were told to press a button for cards with matching name and color (Go). They were instructed to withhold a response (No-Go) when there was a mismatch or when the color name was presented two times in a row. In addition, when the button was erroneously pushed in response to a "No-Go" card, subjects were instructed to push the button a second time to register awareness of their mistake. Before measuring performance, enough practice was allowed to ensure that each person had mastered the instructions. The reason for giving such complex instructions for when *not* to press the button was to intentionally increase the number of errors committed. Ultimately, the test was interested in how aware people are of having committed a mistake.

On average, the regular cannabis users were successful young adults who had used 5–7 days a week for 8 years, after an onset of use at age 16. While users and non-using matched controls committed the same number of errors, non-users were aware of 91 percent of their mistakes, while users were only aware of 77 percent. Reduced awareness of errors limits the ability to improve performance. It is impossible to learn from your mistakes if you lack awareness of them. Given the choice, I think most people would prefer more, not less, error awareness when attempting to improve performance on any task.

Brain imaging conducted during the complex Error Awareness Task revealed an interesting finding. When both users and non-users failed to be aware of their mistake, brain activity was reduced more for users than for non-users in a part of the frontal lobes called the cingulate gyrus. This area tends to be hyperactive in people with obsessive-compulsive disorders, characteristically tormenting them with a false "awareness" of having failed to wash their hands properly or turn off a light correctly. Too much "awareness of error" can be paralyzing. Regular cannabis users experience the opposite – too little activity in the cingulate gyrus and therefore less-than-normal awareness of errors. It should be no surprise that this area of the brain has a dense concentration of CB1 receptors. We need to maintain the proper number of these receptors to have a healthy level of awareness when we make mistakes.

Risk Assessment

People are notoriously bad at understanding statistics. Most have little intuition for how likely or unlikely they are to win the lottery or draw an inside straight in poker. This lack of sense for statistical probabilities can have a real-life impact when it comes to deciding how fast to drive a car or choosing which investments are likely to pay off well. The Iowa Gambling Task was created to measure our capacity to assess risk and reward. The test involves four stacks of cards, each card representing the gain or loss of an amount of money. Some stacks have cards with large gains and losses, and other stacks contain smaller amounts. Participants are told that some stacks produce a better net gain than others, but they are given no clues as to which are good or bad stacks. They are asked to choose cards one at a time from any stack to try to maximize their earnings. A running total of their overall gain or loss is displayed throughout the test. Consistently turning over cards in the high-gain/high-loss stacks ultimately results in net loss, but consistently sticking to the less-exciting stacks that contain smaller amounts results in net gain. The Iowa Gambling Task measures an individual's capacity to assess risk and reward accurately, and thus to favor long-term over short-term gains.

It should probably come as no surprise, as I am including these data, that regular cannabis users did significantly worse than non-using matched controls, meaning lower net gains due to a tendency to choose high-gain/high-loss stacks despite their lower net scores. However, what may be most surprising is that the cannabis users were tested 25 days into a period of abstinence. Given a second trial, users showed less improvement than non-users. When the group of cannabis users was divided by amount of usage (moderate versus heavy), only the heavy users showed lower scores than the control group. Brain imaging revealed lower levels of activity in the frontal lobes of users, with heavy users having less activity than moderate users. Researchers explained the deficit in decision-making in heavy cannabis users as resulting from focusing on the "hit" of high gains while ignoring losses, as if losses are a "mistake" that they paid less attention to.

Our ECS is intimately involved in reducing memories of unpleasant events, which can offer another explanation for the poorer performance of cannabis users in the Iowa Gambling Task. This function was proven by clever classical conditioning experiments. The prototypical classical conditioning experiment trained dogs to salivate in response to a bell by first pairing the bell with a tasty treat. Classical conditioning occurs with both positive reinforcement (e.g. food) and negative reinforcement (e.g. an electric shock). Once the treat is no longer given, dogs continue salivating at the sound of the bell until they finally learn that no more treats are coming. This process of undoing a classically conditioned behavior is called "extinction." In a study of THC's impact on the extinction of negative conditioning, mice learned to jump over a barrier to the other side of their cage when a bell warned of an incoming electric shock to the floor of the side they were currently in. Once the shock stopped following the bell, the time before mice stopped reacting with fear was measured. While THC has no impact on the extinction of classical conditioning that uses positive reinforcement, extinction of negative conditioning happens significantly faster with THC on board. Increasing activity in the ECS shortens the time for extinction of negatively conditioned behavior, and reducing endocannabinoid activity by administering a cannabinoid blocker (rimonabant) lengthens the time required to extinguish negative conditioning. In other words, our ECS eases the forgetting of painful memories. It is a balm that prevents the accumulation of trauma. This is why so many military veterans gravitate toward cannabis to relieve their symptoms of PTSD.

A third reason for poor performance on the Iowa Gambling Task's assessment of risk and reward is revealed in brain imaging conducted in the early stages of the test, when people are first developing a strategy. Everyone begins the Iowa Gambling Task equally unsure which stacks are best. However, non-users display greater activation of the cingulate gyrus, and thus greater error awareness in response to losses (i.e. mistakes). The increased awareness that losses are errors helps mold their strategy. Cannabis users lack this awareness and are slower and less effective in developing a winning strategy. The bottom line is that failure to respond to and remember loss is more important than being overly attracted to gains in explaining the impact of regular cannabis use on risk assessment. Loss needs to be felt if risks are to be assessed properly. The lack of response to loss is part of the destressing and "chill" that cannabis provides. In the end, however, being too chill prevents learning from our losses and mistakes. As the saying goes, "No pain, no gain." Being chill is a choice, but there is not a choice about suffering the consequences of pharmacological serenity – a slowing of learning from hard-won experience, growth, and maturation.

If regular use of cannabis reduces your capacity to be aware of errors, assess risk, and demonstrate sound judgment and effective decision-making by a mere 5 percent, the change would likely not be noticeable. But suffering this 5 percent deficit over several years would represent a subtle fork in the road. At first, the deviation from the trajectory your full capacity would follow is slight. But over time, the effect multiplies until you are headed in a distinctly different direction with different possible outcomes. You are free to take whichever life path you wish, but it is best to be aware of a fork in the road instead of only becoming aware of the consequences of your choice in retrospect.

Robert was distressed by what he learned about the impact of long-term cannabis use on memory and risk assessment. He told me the customer who objected to the extra delivery charge said Robert had tried to add this charge once before. Robert had forgotten this detail, which only added to his misperception of the risk in adding the extra charge. He began to worry that perhaps he was not as accurate at perceiving the tolerable price point for his customers as he imagined himself to be.

Emotion

Some of my favorite cannabis research has looked at the impact of regular use on our emotional life and the role of our ECS in determining the temperament we inherit from our parents. Research in these two areas has produced some of the most intriguing perspectives on the role of cannabinoids in our daily lives. Our focus turns now to the amygdala, one in each hemisphere, often referred to as the emotional center of the brain. Although this is an oversimplification, it is certainly true that the amygdala plays a central role in adding emotional coloring to our lives, as well as being the switchboard that triggers fight and flight reactions when danger is felt.

The amygdala's role in our emotional life undergoes a transition following puberty as the frontal lobes develop. When prepubescent children are shown pictures of human faces with different emotional expressions, MRIs show strong activation of the amygdala. Coincidentally, children are more likely to misinterpret worried expressions as anger. MRI studies conducted a few years later, after puberty has started, reveal that human emotional expressions begin activating both the frontal lobes and the amygdala, and worried expressions are more accurately identified. By late adolescence, there is balanced activation in both the amygdala and the more neurologically mature frontal lobes. This balance permits us to have greater discernment of emotional responses within the larger context of our frontal lobes' ability to support abstract thinking. Thus, it can be seen why frontal lobotomies return people to a more childlike emotional state, and why delayed maturation of the frontal cortex from regular cannabis use during adolescence also delays the psychological maturation of emotional life.

A masked faces protocol has been used to study the reaction to angry facial expressions in adults with a history of regular cannabis use. In masked faces research, fMRIs of the amygdala are recorded while a series of happy and fearful faces are subliminally flashed before a neutral face appears for a longer time. Test subjects are instructed to do nothing but watch the screen, and they remain unaware of the fleeting subliminal images. Brain imaging reveals that the amygdala is activated by subliminal exposure to the angry face in non-users, even though there is no conscious awareness of its presence. This fMRI result is like manna from heaven for a psychiatrist, as it is literally a photograph of the unconscious. It reveals that the brain can process an emotional stimulus beneath the level of conscious awareness – the very definition of the unconscious. Interestingly, no such activation occurs in the amygdala of regular cannabis users. This means regular users process emotional stimuli differently from non-users. More accurately, regular use of cannabis limits the brain's ability to respond to subtle emotional cues. Again, this is part of the "chill" many users covet. In the words of Pink Floyd, they are "comfortably numb."

One of the chief complaints made by spouses of regular cannabis users is that being high robs their partner of emotional presence. I have frequently heard a frustrated spouse try to explain to their partner what is missing, only to be met with incomprehension. As the user's brain is not registering subtle emotional cues, they have no way of understanding what their partner is trying to describe. Again, Pink Floyd illustrated an exaggerated version of the dilemma faced by frustrated spouses:

> *Hello?*
> *Is there anybody in there?*
> *Just nod if you can hear me.*
> *Is there anyone home?*
> "Comfortably Numb," from Pink Floyd's 1979 album, *The Wall.*

This information about insensitivity to emotional cues shook Robert to his core. He stared for a while at the fMRI showing the missing activity in the amygdala of cannabis users, and then asked if this was possibly what his wife meant when she complained he was not fully present. I said it probably was. Furthermore, I wondered if he had missed the first subtle cues that his customer did not like the extra delivery charge. He wondered if a decrease in emotional intelligence was jeopardizing his professional success. Even a slight decrease would be intolerable for him.

Temperament: Introverts and Extroverts

The study of temperament is fascinating because it reveals that many of the tendencies that define us are inherited more than learned or chosen. The genes we inherit determine much of our temperament, such as whether we are introverted or extroverted, and whether our energy cycle peaks early or late in the day. Temperamental differences in our response to novelty have been found to stem from genetically determined differences in the density of CB1 receptors in the amygdala. A lower level of CB1 receptor functionality leads to a lower response to novelty, and thus to a greater attraction to finding novel stimuli. This leads to a less constrained, novelty-seeking personality, which can contribute to both curiosity and impulsivity. In contrast, a high level of CB1 functionality in the amygdala leads to a greater response to novelty and a more constrained, cautious temperament designed to avoid being overwhelmed by too much novel stimulation. We have no more choice over CB1 levels in our amygdala than we do over our height or the color of our eyes. The degree of our novelty seeking and impulsivity is biologically determined. Our task is to manage the temperament we are given and to discover the benefits available from the level of constraint we may or may not have. Different rewards come from being cautious or more impulsive.

What interests me now is whether regular cannabis use alters temperament by chronically downregulating receptors. We already know that regular use reduces the number of CB1 receptors in the amygdala to roughly the variation that occurs genetically. It is unlikely that low CB1 levels induced by cannabis mirror those from genetic variations. It is one thing to experience a reduction in CB1 receptors in the amygdala later in life, and quite another to have this reduced number since conception and throughout brain development and maturation. We cannot expect the two different circumstances to be equivalent. It would be interesting to study changes in temperament before and after starting regular cannabis use. Unfortunately, such research will be difficult because we have no way of knowing who will eventually use cannabis heavily.

Impulsivity

The question of whether people who use cannabis regularly are more impulsive does not have a simple answer. It has long been known that people with an inherent tendency toward novelty seek exposure to more risk. High novelty seeking is a predictor of greater drug use, including cannabis. On average, cannabis users will score higher on tests of impulsivity for reasons that predate their use, and questionnaires measuring impulsivity show that regular cannabis users score higher than non-using matched controls. However, MRIs in regular users with high impulsivity scores also show disruptions in the axons connecting frontal lobes and between areas within each frontal lobe. THC's impact on microtubules interferes with the normal, one-way flow of water found in healthy axons. This disruption decreases the efficiency of communication between nerve cells needed to coordinate brain activity. As a result, cannabis further increases impulsivity in regular users.

Motivation

People have touted amotivation syndrome as a symptom of excessive cannabis use, but I have always had trouble with this concept. I have watched many adolescents abandon their normal pursuits after discovering cannabis, but no one has shown me how to objectively measure motivation. The Gestalt therapist Fritz Perls was said to have asked people to demonstrate they were trying to drop a pillow. After multiple contortions while still holding onto the pillow, it became apparent that motivation is an elusive concept, impossible to see or directly measure. Instead of thinking in terms of amotivation, I consider the boredom and loss of interest in activities that characterizes many regular users to be a failure to respond to novelty. When nothing is novel, people are less likely to be interested and feel motivated in any particular direction, except perhaps to use cannabis again. In addition, when people enter Cannabis Culture, they often begin looking at the world through a different lens. Changing values and aspirations can withdraw interest from pursuits that no longer hold the same meaning.

I was familiar with research showing how rats given THC become "slackers," more likely to choose low-effort/low-reward tasks instead of the high-effort/high-reward tasks they previously pursued. But it was a clever human study that began to change my mind. A delayed monetary reward study asked college students to press a button when a stimulus appeared on the screen. They were promised either $0.20 or $5.00 after the test, depending on their performance. MRI of the reward center was conducted during the test, which was administered at ages 20, 22, and 24. Over the 4 years, those whose cannabis use increased the most were found to have decreasing activation of the reward center in anticipation of financial reward. This interesting research suggests that, as cannabis alters the brain's reward center, regular users begin to anticipate less reward from non-cannabis sources. Cannabis alters the structure and function of reward circuitry to shift attention and priorities away from previous targets and toward cannabis. This is a prime example of the brain being hijacked; the promise of financial gain began stimulating less activity in their reward center. This study shows how the reward for non-cannabis events is lessened as the reward for cannabis increases. Perhaps the couch lock seen in the heaviest cannabis users is not simply a matter of decreased spontaneous motor activity but also results from the brain's inability to signal reinforcing rewards for anything that is not cannabis related. Motivation depends upon the anticipation of reward, and an amotivational syndrome could result from the absence of anticipating reward from anything not involving cannabis.

Psychosis

Introduced in Chapter 9, the topic of psychotic reactions to cannabis, development of schizophrenia from cannabis use, and the impact of cannabis use in schizophrenics is highly charged for many people. The anguish of parents who have watched their child descend into profoundly disabling delusions and hallucinations after using cannabis are heartrending. To them, the cause-and-effect relationship between cannabis and psychosis is clear and certain. Anyone denying that cannabis can cause schizophrenia is seen as a dangerous enemy. In contrast, cannabis advocates rail against unvalidated testimonials that cannabis causes schizophrenia, and many cautious scientists are only comfortable concluding that the two are associated. Because psychosis and schizophrenia are relatively uncommon, most families have not been directly affected by it and most people using cannabis are not personally worried about it.

Brief psychotic reactions to high-THC products are different from the disease of schizophrenia. Novice users are more likely to appear in emergency rooms with transient psychosis, more often for panic reactions, especially when edibles are overused. Cannabis can clearly cause panic, paranoia, and psychotic reactions, although only a small percentage of people have severe enough reactions to require emergency care. However, the incidence of emergency room visits for panic, paranoia, and psychosis has risen as states fully legalize cannabis.

Good data support the idea that cannabis use facilitates the onset of schizophrenia. Cannabis users who develop schizophrenia have an onset 6 years earlier than average and experience more severe symptoms. While the rate of schizophrenia in the general public is 1 percent, it is 2 percent in cannabis users and 4 percent among high-potency and early-onset users. How should we think about the relationship between cannabis and schizophrenia?

Schizophrenia is a genetically caused psychotic disease. There is no single gene that causes schizophrenia but rather a collection of genes that create an ever-greater risk as an increasing number of genes combine. While research clearly shows cannabis to be associated with schizophrenia, the important question is whether it substantively contributes to the likelihood of developing schizophrenia. Every individual's DNA contains some of these genes, but the unlucky among us carry so many that schizophrenia is inevitable. The people of interest in this discussion are those who carry some schizophrenia genes but not enough for the disease to be inevitable.

They are prone to developing schizophrenia but only if other forces tip the scales.

In a similar fashion, I was prone to the onset of disease; I have a family history of diabetes but had no symptoms myself. Then, when I needed a brief course of steroid treatment to quell inflamed nasal passages, my tendency toward diabetes was uncovered. The metabolic stress arising from steroids tipped the scales, and I have been overtly diabetic ever since. Did steroids "cause" my diabetes? I think not. I was already genetically susceptible to diabetes, and steroids challenged my metabolism in a way that pushed me over the edge. Steroids facilitated development of diabetes. Other medications, or even physical trauma, could have been the precipitating factor instead of the steroids. Similarly, cannabis, especially high-THC cannabis, expedites the development of schizophrenia in individuals who are genetically prone to the disease.

In my clinical work, I do not need to ask parents of a psychotic, cannabis-using adolescent whether they think the pot was responsible for driving their kid off the rails. They are usually convinced beyond any doubt that cannabis is the sole factor making their son or daughter "crazy." Their child feels lost to them, no longer the person they've known since birth, suddenly a stranger inside a familiar body. To paraphrase Pink Floyd, there's someone in their head, but it's not them.

When schizophrenia is diagnosed, it no longer matters whether it would have developed independently or whether cannabis tipped the genetic scales. What matters is a recognition that cannabis is especially problematic for schizophrenics. Unfortunately, I have often heard therapists express reluctance to encourage schizophrenic patients to abstain from cannabis, not wanting to take away "one of their few pleasures." This misguided empathy ignores the fact that schizophrenics who continue to use cannabis experience more relapses, more severe symptoms when they relapse, and more hospitalizations. A common prelude to relapse and hospitalization occurs when antipsychotic medications are stopped in favor of cannabis use. It is not difficult to understand why schizophrenic patients might prefer cannabis to their medication, as antipsychotics typically produce uncomfortable side effects and cannabis is generally more enjoyable. However, the consequences of substituting cannabis for medications that more effectively combat psychosis are steep, both for the individual and for their family. For example, studies show that total brain volume declines over 5 years in all schizophrenics, but the decline is greater in those who use cannabis.

The bottom line is that those susceptible to schizophrenia for underlying genetic reasons are more likely to develop the full-blown mental disorder if they use cannabis, particularly if they begin use at an early age, use heavily, and use high-THC products with low CBD. Individuals who develop schizophrenia, whether induced by cannabis or not, would be well advised to avoid all cannabis use, despite the pleasure it may bring.

Conclusion

In addition to the possibility of addiction, regular cannabis use causes a variety of negative impacts on cognition, psychology, emotion, and behavior. Careful research has documented impairments in memory, executive functions, error awareness, assessment of risk and reward, emotional sensitivity, temperament, impulsivity, motivation, and the risk of psychotic illness, including schizophrenia. These research findings are inconvenient truths for anyone using cannabis recreationally or medicinally, as well as for the cannabis industry. These data provide ample ammunition for opponents of liberalizing cannabis policies, but none of these consequences are inevitable, with the possible exception of schizophrenia in people with serious genetic vulnerability. The impairments described above should be thought of as the equivalents of alcoholic liver disease and dementia, albeit far less severe. The vast majority of alcohol users avoid serious impairments, just as the vast majority of cannabis users can prevent potential impairments by avoiding too-frequent use.

As cognitive testing and brain imaging technology improve, researchers hunt for increasingly subtle impacts from smaller and less-frequent cannabis use. The question then becomes, "What constitutes too-frequent use?" Is it daily use? Three times a week? Once a week? Once or twice a month? Unfortunately, there is no cookie-cutter answer that fits everyone. Some researchers define heavy use as 10–19 days a month, with regular use being 20 or more days a month. These distinctions are confused by the fact that the more frequently individuals use cannabis, the larger the quantity they tend to use each time.

Without scientific results to point to, only two answers can be given to the question of how much cannabis use is too much. The first answer requires rigorous self-honesty, and the second requires transparency. First, as every individual has his or her own unique brain and psychology, we each have a different limit. Knowing your limit begins with understanding the five early signs of cannabinoid receptor downregulation that occur when no longer high. Restlessness, anxiety/irritability, boredom, decreased appetite, and insomnia are the earliest warning signs – the canaries in the coal mine. Rigorous honesty with oneself about the appearance of any of these five signs is hard. It takes courage to acknowledge the truth of what is happening to us against our will. Rigorous honesty lies at the core of the Alcoholics Anonymous program because it is essential to living a life of integrity. Unfortunately, the impacts of regular cannabis use erode our ability to maintain honest self-assessment. Too-frequent cannabis use keeps us from remembering its adverse effects, impairs assessment of the risks of regular use, makes it difficult to shift from seeing cannabis as the answer to life's problems to seeing it as the underlying cause of these problems, reduces sensitivity to subtle emotional cues, and diminishes our motivation for things unrelated to cannabis.

Second, because the effects of regular cannabis use work against rigorous self-honesty, transparency is necessary. It is important to be open to hearing the observations and opinions of trusted family and friends, including those who are outside Cannabis Culture. If you are hiding your use, minimizing it to others, or sneaking more than those around you realize, you are keeping yourself opaque. Why? Perhaps you fear their judgment. If so, you should seek out someone, even a professional, whom you can trust to give you an objective, non-judgmental perspective on whether your use is having impacts you cannot see for yourself. Transparency also takes courage. It is difficult to hear something negative about ourselves without becoming defensive. Transparency is hard work that requires diligent and persistent effort.

In the end, we are all free to do what we please. We are free to agree with someone else's opinion or not, and we are free to continue using anyway. But not being aware of the five signs of using too frequently or the consequences of regular use robs us of being able to make truly well-informed choices. The slogan "Know Your Limits" expresses an important goal, but merely knowing your limits is not enough. It is only by staying within these limits that we maintain wellness and balance.

After listening carefully to what I had to say, Robert looked sad. He said his wife must not be as crazy as he had thought. She may have been overreacting a little, but she had a good point. He promised to put his marijuana away for 3 months to see if anything changed, although he knew he would miss it. Robert decided not to tell his wife about his abstinence for a while and would eventually ask if she saw any change. He thought of himself as conducting an experiment to gather information about the impact of his use. I said I admired his commitment to being honest with himself and his openness to his wife's input.

Perhaps he was reaching a new fork in the road.

14 TREATMENT AND RECOVERY

Monique was charming, restless, independent, and willful. Always surrounded by friends, she was the adventurous risk-taker among them. Quick-witted, Monique liked to learn but not to be taught. Her body developed early, writing checks that her mind was unprepared to cash. Older boys quickly targeted her when she entered high school, and with the boys came their drugs, tobacco, and alcohol. She started with cannabis.

Monique sought the boys' attention by sneaking out at night and enthusiastically joining in with their drug use. Her parents tried to talk to Monique about their concerns, but her ears were shut and she complained that her parents were control freaks. Unsure whether Monique was just going through a wild phase or if this was the prelude to disaster, her parents saw that she had stopped giving them any authority and consulted a therapist for guidance.

When deciding whether to consider treatment for excessive cannabis use, two questions are prudent to ask. First, is cannabis causing or intensifying problems in the user's life? To state the obvious, people have a drug problem when the drug is causing problems. As the previous chapter illustrated, ongoing, regular cannabis use can interfere with school and work performance, financial independence, and the ability to maintain healthy relationships, especially with an intimate partner. It is never easy to know for sure whether cannabis is directly causing a given problem, and a period of abstinence is the only way to find out.

Second, is the person able to stop using cannabis for a significant period of time, preferably 3–6 months? This is long enough to determine (1) if symptoms of withdrawal occur, (2) if problems improve, and (3) whether the quality of life without cannabis improves. Unwillingness to experiment with a trial of cannabis-free life is often a sign that addiction is present, and the possibility of addiction needs to be explored. Failure to maintain abstinence throughout an intended trial period suggests that a recovery process may be necessary to develop a satisfying level of improvement.

When cannabis use has become problematic and a person has difficulty establishing abstinence, a course of treatment can help. If therapy were not stigmatized as much as it is, seeking treatment would sound as sensible as asking your doctor to treat your hypertension. But both drug abuse and drug treatment are very often a source of embarrassment and shame. Additionally, most people who are harmfully involved with cannabis are deeply ambivalent about stopping their use and are therefore quite resistant to thoughts of treatment.

The principles of cannabis treatment are simple and do not differ substantially from treating any other drug dependence. In the early stages of abstinence, people need basic education about cannabis, its impact on their brain and psychology, and the skills needed to avoid relapse. Sometimes medication needs to be prescribed to help people tolerate withdrawal. Education about how to live without the balm and distraction of cannabis is essential. Perhaps most importantly, people entering recovery need enough welcoming and non-judgmental support to instill hope for a better future. Others who have successfully established a drug-free life can often communicate this hope more believably than even the best professional counselor. Because they have been there, they can offer a realistic, first-hand view of what changes in lifestyle and beliefs are needed to lead a satisfying life without cannabis. This process of learning to live life on life's terms is generally called recovery. Any underlying mental health issues also need to be identified and treated with therapy and medication, when necessary. When people are past the stage of physical withdrawal, the goal of addiction treatment is to remove any barriers standing in the way of working a strong program of recovery. This work involves an increasing commitment to emotional growth and honesty with oneself and others.

Although the elements of treatment and recovery are not complex, the work they require is very hard, for both those in recovery and those who treat them. The work is hard for professionals because it is impossible to directly control the minds and behavior of the people they want to help. On the surface, addiction treatment seems different from surgery or the rest of medicine, where you can cut out the problem or prescribe an antibiotic to cure infection. However, doctors and nurses are often frustrated by their inability to control whether people fully cooperate with their prescribed treatment. One patient may not finish physical rehab after their hip replacement or may fail to lose weight as directed. Another may stop an antibiotic as soon as they feel better and then return to work too early. The reality is that virtually all medical treatments will only be partially successful if patients don't make the lifestyle and behavioral changes needed to sustain good health. When alcohol or other drug use stands in the way of recovering physical health, many doctors surrender the fight and feel impotent to make a difference. It is a simple fact that people have difficulty changing entrenched behaviors, whether this entails alcohol and drugs, overeating, underexercising, overworking, or ignoring the level of stress in their lives. Treating addiction must deal with the normal human resistance to change, but it is further complicated because excessive drug and alcohol use modify the brain by hijacking the reward system and bending motivation toward continued drug use. It takes specialized training and unique personal characteristics to effectively treat someone addicted to any drug, including cannabis. Treatment providers must possess the capacity to remain optimistic about anyone's ability to recover, despite having seen too many fine and lovely people resist changing, much to their own detriment. With drugs harder than cannabis, especially alcohol and opiates, resistance to change is too often fatal. Treatment professionals must also possess a truly non-judgmental attitude, a genuine curiosity about other people's subjective experiences, and the willingness and ability to engage empathically with people who are suffering. They must also be comfortable with having only the power to influence rather than control others. Many of these characteristics are simply part of a counselor's basic temperament and are difficult to teach.

What makes "living life on life's terms" a worthwhile goal? Isn't this the wolf of moral judgment wrapped in therapeutic sheep's clothing? Isn't most of America and the world at large already committed to "better living through chemistry," whether it's a couple of nightly drinks, Xanax, Prozac, and/or hits of cannabis? After all, someone taking Prozac to treat disabling depression would be right to resist stopping the medication. Uncomfortable symptoms may occur when they discontinue Prozac and depression may worsen. It would be foolish to stop a medicine that their mental and emotional health depends upon. For many people, the line between taking medication to treat a diagnosed psychiatric condition and using a socially accepted drug to feel better is fuzzy and difficult to distinguish.

With all this complexity in mind, what would make a drug-free life desirable? Rather than debate this question in the abstract, I will approach it pragmatically. All medications and self-administered drugs have possible benefits and potential side effects. It is especially difficult for the consumer to evaluate the risk:benefit ratio of drugs that alter the mind and affect consciousness. Once the mind is altered, the ability to see the full impact of this alteration is affected. This is especially true of any drug that has the addictive potential for changing the very infrastructure in the brain that produces reward and motivation. When this happens, we can become blind to the negative side effects of the medication or drug being consumed. We can become like a blind person who changes their hair color and needs to rely on someone else to give feedback on how it looks. In such a case, it makes sense to ask someone we trust and who has a good sense of style. In a similar way, anyone using a psychoactive medication or drug would be wise to seek observations about its impact from an objective observer, preferably someone with familiarity with the drug's potential benefits and side effects. In the case of Prozac, the watchful eye of a caring doctor is theoretically in place, as it requires a prescription.

Cannabis, in contrast, is a powerful drug that many self-administer. The budista at a local dispensary may have reams of knowledge about each cannabis variety they sell, how it is grown, and the subtle nuances of its high, but they are not trained in cannabis addiction, nor are they tasked with warning people about the potential negative effects of overuse. They should not be expected to protect the public's health any more than the clerk at a liquor store.

Objective Assessment of Cannabis Use

Where can people consuming cannabis turn for an objective assessment of the negative impacts of their use? This is a difficult question to answer. The parents of an adolescent using cannabis are unlikely to be objective. Even if they did reflect objective reality, most teens, and especially teens who are using cannabis frequently, are very unlikely to give their parents' opinion much weight. A spouse's opinion that their partner is being negatively affected by their cannabis use rarely has the wished-for impact. Once a cannabis user adopts the Cannabis Culture perspective, they become less open to the entreaties of anyone they perceive as not understanding, too rigid, moralistic, or judgmental.

If you use cannabis with regularity, I recommend occasional periods of abstinence to assess whether any of the five signs of overuse appear: restlessness, anxiety/irritability, boredom, decreased appetite, and insomnia. It is important to accept that no definitive definition of "regularly" can be given. The definition depends solely on your own brain's unique capacity to maintain normal ECS balance and function. For one person, "regularly" will mean daily or nearly daily. For another, it can mean as little as once a week. Assessing existence of the five signs requires rigorous self-honesty; it can be very easy to excuse even the most obvious signs of downregulation. The best course of action is complete transparency with someone who loves you enough to tell you the truth. When you abstain, do they see increased restlessness, anxiety/irritability, boredom, decreased appetite, or insomnia? Pay special attention to whether they make spontaneous comments about your becoming more present or emotionally available. If you are unwilling to be transparent, is it because you are protecting your cannabis use? What makes its continued use important enough to keep any possible side effects unrecognized and secret?

If any of the five signs appear, you have hard evidence that your use is frequent enough to alter your brain, and therefore your mind, even when you aren't high. Once you acknowledge this reality, there are several questions you might ask yourself. Is this ongoing impact acceptable to you? Have people around you been complaining about the impact of your cannabis use? Are you experiencing problems that reduce your satisfaction with life?

In the end, the best evidence that addiction exists is not just withdrawal, but whether you are able to maintain abstinence. If you relapse before the end of an experimental trial, when and why did you return to using? Was it due to stress or boredom? Or did you simply no longer want to feel negative emotions? Was it due to feeling excluded when friends were getting high and you weren't? Was it because you just liked using cannabis and missed it? Or that it is your main way of having fun? Is it the only way you feel comfortable when alone, or with others? Is it your best way of reducing anxiety? Or your only way of relaxing? Perhaps the most important question is whether being high is substituting for some part of your psychology or spirituality that is undeveloped.

In summary, the way to ensure you are using cannabis safely is the following formula. After you have chosen the length of abstinence, observe (1) if symptoms of withdrawal occur, (2) whether problems improve, (3) whether life gets better without cannabis, and (4) whether you completed the intended period of abstinence. The likelihood that your love of cannabis could bias your perception of any improvement requires transparency with a partner or trusted friend during the trial of abstinence to achieve objectivity. If you learn from this trial that treatment might be useful, there is one more step to take before arriving at this conclusion: seek consultation with an addiction specialist. If you sense that a mental health issue may also be present, it would be best to consult with an addiction specialist who has wider medical or mental health expertise than addiction alone.

What can be expected from an assessment with an addiction specialist? First, you should expect to learn whether your self-assessment is accurate. Have you over- or under-estimated the severity and importance of what you discovered during your abstinence trial? In addition, you will learn how it feels to talk honestly with someone familiar with drug experience and learn more about the nature of addiction. And finally, you should expect to learn about resources for help that exist in your area. Many people assume that treatment automatically means 28 days away from home and work in a residential facility. This is rarely the case for cannabis, especially for adults. The full range of treatment and recovery options includes attendance at 12-step meetings (Marijuana Anonymous, where available), individual counseling, outpatient programs designed around school or work schedules, and more intensive residential treatment programs. When you leave the assessment, you should know the paths available to you, have a recommendation for which option best fits your needs, and be free to choose which ones, if any, you want to pursue. Throughout the entire self-examination and consultation process, you will never lose your right to decide what is best for yourself. However, you might gain enough new information and insight to recognize that it would be best to change your cannabis use. At this point, the real work begins.

I have often heard it said that no one enters treatment voluntarily. Whether it is under court order, at the demand of a partner or parent, or simply a recognition of previously denied realities of one's life, nearly everyone enters treatment because they have to, not because they necessarily want to. Resistance to seeking medical care is commonly found in a variety of medical conditions, from unexplained weight loss and low energy to gradually increasing hip pain. The first reactions to the possibility of illness are often denial, soldiering on as if nothing serious is happening, and an effort to suppress fear. All of these reactions, but especially denial, are often found to an exaggerated degree in addiction. Motivation to continue using is entrenched and heightened by drug-induced changes in the brain's reward center. This physically driven motivation bends a person's psychology toward defending drug use and denying the downsides of overuse. To a hijacked reward center, more is better, and more further hijacks the brain.

Denial

People generally resist seeing themselves, or being seen by others, as misusing alcohol or drugs. Once the possibility of a problem is acknowledged, the specter of change and loss of pleasure is raised. When faced with facts that are too uncomfortable to accept, people often insist the facts are not true, despite overwhelming evidence to the contrary. This unwillingness to admit the obvious is called denial. Sometimes, denial is a conscious suppression of the truth, and sometimes it runs so deeply that a person is wholly unconscious of what they are denying. In any case, denial is baffling and very frustrating to family, friends, and co-workers. The skill of addiction treatment professionals lies in their ability to develop deep enough relationships with addicted individuals to identify, discuss, and work through their multiple levels of denial to arrive at truths they can no longer avoid.

It is critically important to understand two aspects of denial that are not immediately apparent. First, sometimes denial results from drug-induced cognitive impairment. As shown in Chapter 13, deficits in frontal-lobe executive functions can look like denial. When someone is using enough cannabis to lower their scores on the Wisconsin Card Sort's test of the ability to shift nimbly between points of view, they may also lack the ability to shift easily from seeing cannabis as the answer to their problems to seeing it as the cause of these problems. While this may look like an unwillingness to admit the obvious, it may also be partially due to a cognitive glitch that reduces mental flexibility. This fact underlies addiction professionals' view that addiction is a brain disorder.

Second, the classic understanding of denial is that it occurs *unconsciously*. Recall how MRIs revealed activity in the amygdala when non-users were exposed to subliminal photos of fearful faces. This research provided a picture of brain activity while test participants remained completely unconscious of both the stimulus and the early gestation of their emotional response. The brain is pervasively active in a universe of ways that never achieve consciousness – emotions, thoughts, beliefs, biases, predilections, desires, values, and more. No one knows how consciousness ultimately occurs as a result of all this brain activity, but we do know it is absent when the brain is fully anesthetized. Somehow, out of all the swirling neural activity, consciousness emerges. Perhaps each neuron is sentient in its own limited way. With enough communication among all the neurons in the brain, the quality of consciousness is born.

The surfacing of consciousness from the highly inter-connected network of living neurons is a natural phenomenon, and not mystical. It is similar to how a generational identity emerges among highly interconnected humans or how a community forms among people recovering from addiction. When a group consciousness emerges and plays back on individuals within that group, it changes their behavior. In the case of people recovering from addiction, inclusion in the recovering community feeds back on each person's emotions and thoughts about sobriety. This process of group awareness is how neural activity combines to produce the emergent quality we call consciousness. This consciousness is not contained in any individual neuron, but it does play back on neurons to modify the amount and meaning of their activity. Altering neural activity with cannabis results in the emergence of a different quality of consciousness than is normally experienced, and this cannabis-induced altered consciousness can contribute to denial.

Beneath the level of consciousness, fears and desires can block our ability to view reality objectively, and this may be particularly true in regard to self-observations. Denial operates as an unconscious filter in the mind. When denial filters out awareness of cannabis dependence, the mind naturally manufactures a host of "reasons," explanations, rationalizations, and minimizations to make sense of or excuse cannabis use. Denial of addiction also leads to blaming other people, places, and things for one's problems, when these problems actually have their roots in excessive cannabis use. The denial of cannabis addiction is often so blatant that family and friends have difficulty responding with cool reason and warm empathy. Instead, out of their frustration and inability to understand the user's experience, family and friends may become irritable and unreasonable, often without realizing how exaggerated and ineffective their reactions are becoming. Tension, anger, and hostility creep into the behavior of all involved, disrupting normal relationships. Unhappiness descends on the family as everyone's posture hardens. Blame and self-protection begin to dominate interactions as the family unit itself becomes less functional. The denial of problems caused by cannabis exists along a continuum, from mild defensiveness to a total inability to see the truth about oneself. I have seen people at all points along this continuum in my practice.

The percentage of people seeking treatment for cannabis rose as the potency of cannabis flowers and products increased. Some adolescent treatment facilities now report that the majority of admissions are specifically for CUD. In most cases, it is not the adolescent who seeks treatment. Approximately half of the treatment for adolescent CUD is forced by the juvenile justice system. The other half is initiated by parents who no longer feel capable of dealing with the issue themselves.

How to Help

How can family and friends recognize when treatment would be useful for someone they love and feel responsible for? When is it time to intervene? And how should parents intervene?

First, educate yourself, as Monique's parents did by meeting with a therapist. Cannabis is a complex plant. People use it for a variety of reasons. Do not rely solely on your own past experience with cannabis or on the opinions of friends unfamiliar with addiction. Be aware that much of the information from news outlets and the Internet is biased and cherry-picked scientific facts to support their position. Dive into literature you can trust to be objective and balanced. Learn the science well, because the person you are concerned about likely knows a lot of cannabis science, much of which has unfortunately been collected from pro-cannabis websites to support use and deny or minimize potential side effects. If you are interested in furthering your education, the Further Reading section of this book contains links to additional information, including reports and journal articles accepted by the scientific community. The links provide access to brief abstracts of important scientific articles at no cost to the public through the federally sponsored PubMed website.

Second, examine yourself and the behavior you model around drugs and alcohol. There is no surer way to under-cut your message of concern about your child's cannabis use than hypocrisy. Are you in a healthy relationship with medication, tobacco, alcohol, and recreational drugs, or do you use pharmacology to replace psychological skills you neglected to develop? Monique's parents eliminated the bottle of wine they routinely bought each weekend. They never drank to intoxication, but they did realize that the wine was used to celebrate the end of their work week and as a lubricant for beginning the weekend's relaxation. Although they felt their drinking was doing no harm to themselves, they realized that it was not the right behavior to model for a daughter who was recklessly using alcohol and cannabis.

Third, I strongly urge you to attend at least a few Al-Anon meetings. Al-Anon provides an opportunity to meet and learn from others in your community who contend with the same issues you face. There is hard-won wisdom in Al-Anon that can provide a useful perspective on how your efforts to control someone's drug use can inadvertently inflame a situation rather than calm it. The single most common mistake made when dealing with someone else's addiction is to try to control them through pleading, threatening, punishing, or yelling. The keystone of Al-Anon is to remember the reality of what is truly under your control: only your own behavior. Al-Anon's guiding principles can aid your efforts to support a family member by: (1) respecting their right to think and feel as they choose, (2) maintaining a loving connection despite their continued destructive behavior, (3) being clear about what you see that concerns you and what you hope they will do to recover better health, and (4) setting and maintaining clear boundaries around what behavior you will and will not tolerate. In addition, Al-Anon encourages people to tolerate their own fears while watching someone they love struggle with behavior only they can choose to change. This is very hard work for family, friends, and even counselors and therapists. The more thoroughly you embody Al-Anon principles, the more likely you are to have a beneficial influence on a loved one's cannabis use. While Al-Anon offers no guarantee of success in getting a loved one to stop their destructive behavior, it does offer a promise that its principles will bring greater health and peace to anyone willing to practice them faithfully.

Monique's father immediately resonated with Al-Anon's admission of the impossibility of controlling another person's feelings, beliefs, and behavior. He acknowledged that he had been insisting Monique listen to and obey him. He realized how much he had resented being treated in the same way by his own father. It was no wonder Monique was resisting his control. Her mother attended Al-Anon only intermittently because of the pain and worry she felt when she sat among people who were confronting even more serious problems with their children. Eventually, she connected with a friend she hadn't known was dealing with an older son who had been arrested for a DUI (driving under the influence), and she learned how the program had helped their family navigate that turmoil together.

Fourth, you must wrestle with the concept that "addiction is a brain disorder" and come to terms with whatever truth you can find in this concept. Of course, the decision to experiment with any drug or alcohol is a voluntary act, but the temperament we inherit, especially the degree of risk and novelty we seek, happens to us. No one voluntarily chooses these traits. The speed with which addiction occurs also differs for genetic reasons. No one chooses to have the tendency to become quickly addicted. Then, once addiction begins to hijack the brain, motivation bends toward behaviors that maintain the addiction. No one volunteers to have the structure and function of their brain's reward mechanism altered. Once addiction is established, a person's brain and mind work differently from how they previously did. They understand the world and their behavior through the veil of their addiction. Abstinence and recovery offer the only path back to good brain and mental health. Until this occurs, people with addiction will filter everything you say and do through the perspective of their altered brain. The sheer subtlety of this alteration often makes it hard to see that brain dysfunction of a diaphanous nature lies at the base of their dysfunctional behavior. No voluntary decision can reverse the brain disorder underlying addiction unless it leads to enough abstinence for brain chemistry to return to a healthy balance. Even then, a return to use may quickly reactivate addiction.

Al-Anon's non-judgmental acceptance of addiction as a brain disorder helped Monique's parents move beyond the shame and embarrassment they felt over their daughter's drug problem. The question of what they had done wrong became one of what they could do now.

Fifth, become familiar with treatment resources in your community, including the names of specialists trained in the assessment of addiction. The goal is to be ready to offer help navigating medical insurance issues and finding treatment professionals if and when the person you are concerned about asks for help. This moment is often fleeting, so you want to be ready to provide the needed information immediately. In many cases, the first step will be to make an appointment with a professional who can do a thorough assessment and recommend the next steps. You may even benefit from meeting with a professional yourself to discuss how you can be more influential by adjusting some of your own attitudes and behavior. Monique's parents met with a therapist who only needed one appointment to direct them to Al-Anon and arm them with all the local resources available to their daughter.

Sixth, the approach to helping minors differs from that for helping adults, but the formula for speaking to both is the same. It is important to begin any discussion of your concern about someone's cannabis use with an earnest, unconditional expression of caring for them. Then, you should provide specific and concrete examples of the behaviors that cause you to be concerned. Saying only that someone uses too frequently is easily dismissed as a judgment call, a mere opinion. A more impactful statement would be to recall how their grades fell after starting use, that they lost a job after increasing use, or that familial responsibilities such as doing chores, providing financial support, attending a birthday party, or eating dinner with the family have all been neglected as use increased. While people with addiction could argue that these things are not due to cannabis, they cannot deny that the incidents happened. You and the cannabis user may disagree on the role cannabis plays in creating your concerns, but you can hold onto your view, despite their denial. Of course, you may be wrong, but an assessment by a specialist would be useful for helping everyone gain perspective. A period of abstinence would also be a useful way to sort out the truth. When these suggestions are rejected, you have yet another reason to communicate your concern. Is an inconvenient truth being avoided? Is that why your loved one is unwilling to speak to a professional or to begin a trial of abstinence? These questions present an opportunity to describe what you hope they will do to explore the impact of their use, as well as to explain what help you are willing to provide. Conversations should always be bookended with a declaration of your deep love.

Recovery

It is helpful to remember that the changes required to recover from any addiction are difficult and unrelenting, especially in the early stages of abstinence. In addition, the decision to abstain from an ingrained cannabis habit entails profound loss. People in recovery often have to leave close friends they have known for years. It can be too awkward and dangerous to hang out with old companions who are still using and who actually discourage abstinence. Cannabis itself has been a reliable friend, offering immediate solace and pleasure on demand. I have heard many people in recovery lament being "condemned to awareness," meaning having only one form of consciousness available to them: the straight, natural consciousness stemming from a well-balanced brain. Gone is the other world of a cannabis-induced high. Losing the ability to check in and out of altered consciousness can feel constricting. Recovery offers only one form of consciousness, 24/7, continuous awareness. When boredom, stress, isolation, or sadness is experienced, there is no easy escape. Condemned to awareness, they need to find healthy ways to tolerate the moment and regulate their inner life. To the aficionado of pharmacologically altering consciousness, this can feel like a profound loss of control. Life on life's terms requires more work than simply lighting up a joint. Recovery is hard work. It is also unfair. While many people can take an occasional, temporary vacation from the relentlessness of day-to-day consciousness without falling into the maw of addiction, those prone to addiction quickly find themselves using frequently enough to alter their thinking and emotions, even when not high. Once recovery is chosen, the path that must be followed narrows if a healthy brain and mind are to be maintained. The seduction of pharmacologically altering consciousness is eventually seen as not worth the risk. The rewards of recovery are too great and too hard won to be jeopardized for a few hours of pleasure, especially when those few hours are likely to jump-start the repetitive use characteristic of addiction.

Recovery requires two things: recognition of the impairment and suffering caused by cannabis, and the ability to think through the consequences that inevitably occur with relapse *before* deciding to use. Most people in recovery are helped by being part of a community that continually works to remain aware of the consequences of reactivating an addiction. In a sense, the wisdom of the recovering community shores up each member's ability to remember and think through the consequences of relapse. Membership in the group consciousness enables the individual to remember what they are unable to remember on their own.

Adolescents who are overly attracted to cannabis often lack the experience, cognitive maturity, and supportive community to give much thought to recovery. During the excitement of discovering cannabis, feeling suddenly independent, and the seemingly unlimited ability to transcend the discomforts and awkwardness of no longer being a child but not yet carrying the weight of an adult, adolescents are at the highest risk of diving into unrestrained cannabis use. On average, 15 percent of 12–14-year-olds who begin using cannabis will be addicted within 2 years. Most have not yet experienced enough painful consequences or developed sufficient executive function to understand what is happening to them. Nor are many adolescents surrounded by a community dedicated to recovery. Quite the opposite – while the majority of their peers have not yet experimented with cannabis, the more vocal influencers, social media, and pop culture all promote the value of getting high. The majority of cannabis addiction has a pediatric origin. Adolescents devoted to cannabis tend to be highly resistant to the restrictions of abstinence and recovery, while parents are legally and morally responsible for the health and safety of their minor children. While this situation is a perfect storm for family tension and conflict, it is also an opportunity for early intervention before lasting damage is done.

Intervening in Adolescent Cannabis Use

Intervening in a child's excessive cannabis use is much easier said than done. Many parents fail to see how seriously their child has been captivated by cannabis. Naiveté, shame and embarrassment, or an unwillingness to think poorly of their child's behavior, all contribute to inaction. Parents who experimented with pot or even used it to excess as adolescents often excuse their child's use as a normal phase that will soon be outgrown. I have to remind them that they probably did not begin use as early as their child has, nor did they use cannabis as strong as is available today. They certainly did not vape high-THC concentrate back then. Many are unsure of the proper use of parental authority and boundaries in a time when they expected to be relinquishing the tighter monitoring and control that was appropriate with grade schoolers.

Not every child harmfully involved with cannabis presents the same challenge to their parents. While some youth blatantly announce their conversion to Cannabis Culture by sprouting dreadlocks and wearing T-shirts emblazoned with Bob Marley's image, others become experts at maintaining "normal" behavior, even when very high. Exercising parental responsibility in both of these extremes begins with educating yourself. If you have read this far, you already know a thing or two about cannabis, including the five signs of overuse. Is your child showing increased restlessness, anxiety/irritability, boredom, decreased appetite, or insomnia? These signs often present the first concrete behaviors for concern. Unfortunately, these behaviors can also characterize normal adolescence, except perhaps decreased appetite. Boredom is the default state for many adolescents, especially when around parents rather than friends. However, adolescents using too much cannabis are more likely to show these signs at family gatherings or other times when it is difficult to use secretly. Other signs to watch for involve changes in your child's peer group, academic achievement, and interests. Have friendships changed to include peers who are already known to be using cannabis? Is your child dropping, or being dropped by, friends who do not use cannabis? Have study habits deteriorated? Do teachers report a new lack of interest and class participation? Has participation in sports or other activities that necessarily exclude use begun to wane? Has your child become more secretive? Are they unwilling to hug after getting home from being with friends to hide the telltale odor of smoke? While some of these changes are totally normal during adolescence, they may be the only signs that cannabis has become too important for your child. Taken together, and especially if your child's resistance to parental authority is mounting, it is time to address your concern directly.

Ideally, a healthy relationship to alcohol and other drugs has been an ongoing part of family conversations and was properly modeled since early childhood. When this has not been the case, and especially when a parent's own use of psychoactive substances has been a routine part of their life, beginning a discussion of cannabis with your teenage child can be difficult and awkward for everyone. This is when I like turning an old adage on its head: "If it's worth doing, it's worth doing badly." The bottom line is that the conversation needs to be started, even if it doesn't generate real participation on your child's part or go perfectly. The point is to stick a flag in the ground. Parents have a right to express their values and concerns, and eventually, a right to learn if their child is jeopardizing their health. Of course, you should avoid beginning the conversation in overtly damaging ways, but do not let your sense of uncertainty or awkwardness be a reason to wait months or years. Just don't charge in like a bull in a china shop with accusations, judgments, and a vain belief that you can command your child to think or feel differently. It is far better to approach the conversation as a calm exchange of information. You want to know how your child views cannabis and you want to express your views, especially your specific concerns about use that is too frequent, too much, and too early. In general, listening with curiosity is more effective than talking. Allowing long silences instead of quickly filling them can open enough space for your child to speak more honestly.

The Talk

Remember the simple formula for expressing your concerns, summarized by the following words: care, see, feel, want, will, and care. Start by expressing the bond you feel with your child and explain how much you care about them. This sets a gentle tone. Be clear and concrete about the behavior you have observed. Describe how it has felt to see the things that concern you. Tell your child what you want for them – honesty, openness, caution with cannabis, and good health, for example. Depending on the seriousness of the situation, you may want your child to delay, reduce, or completely stop their use. State what you are willing to do to help your child make these changes. This can range from help with study habits and transportation to healthier activities to finding a counselor or therapist for your child. The conversation needs to end with further emphasis on your care, love, and hopes for their long-term health and happiness. Care, see, feel, want, will, and care.

Monique's parents felt good about their talk with her. She had initially been silent and sullen. When she finally spoke, she had defended herself by minimizing the risks. Finally, she accused her parents of being the most controlling people in town. But her parents never took the bait. Their tone remained calm, even as they acknowledged their frustration. They could see that their concern had an impact on Monique, although only time would reveal whether anything would change.

Contracting

When conversations don't go well or when they don't lead to change, it is time to enter another phase: contracting. The goal of contracting is to make it increasingly difficult for a child to continue using cannabis, or to get them into treatment if they remain unwilling to comply with a contract they have agreed to. When a child is willing to enter into a contract, the process happens in stages. Contracts are written, signed, and copies are given to all participants. They spell out the steps you want your child to take and the privileges you are willing to provide if the contract is kept. For example, in order for your child to have the privilege of spending the night at a friend's house, you may want the names and phone numbers of the friend's parents to discuss the need for a supervised, drug-free environment. You may provide a tutor for difficult subjects and ask your child to share homework assignments and grades with you on a regular basis in subjects where their grades have fallen. You may want your child's bedroom door left ajar in order to monitor for the odor of burning marijuana, and in exchange, you will continue to provide a cell phone. In some cases, you may want total abstinence from cannabis, which your child can document with saliva testing. If they cooperate, you can offer the privilege of receiving an allowance. An excellent resource for learning more about contracting is included in the Further Reading section. Failure to adhere to an agreed-upon period of cannabis abstinence, or their refusal to sign a contract calling for abstinence, should result in a professional assessment. Be clear from the start that failure to remain abstinent will be interpreted as an inability rather than merely a choice. Contracting combines carrots and sticks. It also provides your child with some autonomy to make their own decisions about how much to cooperate within the boundaries you have set. In the end, however, parents have the right to keep their home free of cannabis use.

Monique resisted contracting with her parents, even after losing her cell phone privileges. It was only when her parents announced they were arranging admission to a residential treatment program that Monique agreed to a contract. The contract included oral drug testing at both random intervals and for cause. When Monique failed a cannabis test a month later, she cooperated with the consequence she had agreed to earlier: assessment by a qualified therapist. The assessment turned into ongoing counseling as the therapist engaged Monique in discussing her long-term goals. Over time, she understood how her behavior was jeopardizing her goal of attending college and law school, which she successfully completed 3 years ago, cannabis and alcohol free.

When I perform an assessment of an adolescent's cannabis use, I always begin by exploring in detail what they like about getting high. I explain that the experience is not the same for everyone and I want to know what they notice and value most about being high. Then I ask what they know about how cannabis produces the experiences they enjoy. When I can engage an adolescent in learning more about how cannabis works, I can usually connect with them over my own fascination with brain science. As they become more confident that I am not attacking their attraction to cannabis, we can freely discuss how much is known about this amazing plant. In the process, I can begin introducing the inconvenient truths about receptor down-regulation, the five signs of using too frequently, and, eventually, addiction. My goal is to be seen as trustworthy, non-judgmental, well informed, and caring, which ultimately increases their willingness to accept enough information about the potential side effects of cannabis to generate uncertainty in their position. Their willingness to realistically weigh the rewards and costs of early-onset cannabis use is not the result of forcing my old-man opinions on them. Rather, it stems from my respecting their experience and their ability to make healthy decisions when armed with all the facts. Not every adolescent is willing to enter into a meaningful conversation with the approach I have just described, but most do. Those who willfully continue using cannabis risk being forced into treatment before their 18th birthday if their parents become desperate enough to exercise their full legal authority. Alternatively, parents with sufficient resources frequently arrange to have their recalcitrant child escorted to wilderness programs capable of isolating adolescents for long enough to withdraw them from cannabis and elicit their cooperation to attend a therapeutic boarding school. This approach is far more expensive than the vast majority of families can afford. In many cases, such extreme measures would not be necessary if an adequate adolescent treatment system existed locally.

America's Missing Adolescent Treatment System

Programs for youth prevention and treatment should begin in schools, the "workplace" for almost every child. Well-funded Student Assistance Programs (SAPs), modeled after Employee Assistance Programs, educate teachers on recognizing early signs of drug use and mental health issues, and offer basic counseling to students in a confidential setting. SAPs also conduct ongoing parental drug education and foster a recovery-sensitive atmosphere within the student body. Counselors track students with drug-related problems during summer vacations and prepare incoming high-school students to meet the challenges of an environment with greater drug availability and use. When counselors sense that a thorough medical/

psychiatric assessment and possible treatment is needed, they should be able to refer students to a local outpatient clinic that serves nearby schools. Rural areas may need to rely more heavily on telehealth services.

Local clinics need to coordinate with schools to maintain students' educational progress, including scheduling assessments and treatment programs after school hours and assuring transportation is provided. Full medical/psychiatric evaluations should then determine the level of drug education and treatment needed for each student, including offering groups focused on trauma, family dysfunctions, and other special needs in order to remove barriers to recovery. Although a variety of different group strategies have been developed, research has found that they all produce roughly the same results. In the end, a therapist's skill and empathy are probably more important than the particular treatment strategy used. Clinics for adolescents should be physically separate from adult treatment programs in order to protect vulnerable youth from improper advances and to maintain focus on age-appropriate developmental issues. Clinic staff with special expertise in outreach should maintain relationships with treatment dropouts and pursue homeless youth and school dropouts in need of drug assessment and treatment. A higher level of training is required for staff in youth treatment than for those working in adult treatment; youth counselors must know how to respond to the rapid psychological development characteristic of adolescence and meet the immediate needs of family therapy, endeavoring to improve the home environment for youth in recovery.

In a small number of cases, either because sufficient abstinence cannot be maintained or because the home environment is too dangerously toxic, referral to a residential setting serving multiple outpatient clinics will be necessary. Coordination with local clinics and schools must be a high priority in order to reintegrate students back into lower levels of treatment intensity as soon as possible. The goal should always be to keep making educational progress, a critically important path for stepping successfully into adulthood. Ultimately, the time available for adolescent development is limited. The patient's 18th birthday will come inevitably, and ready or not, they will be freed from the legal obligation to attend school, participate in treatment, or live with a parent or guardian. Time is short, so intervening early to provide treatment opportunities when they can be most effective must be a high priority.

Conclusion

Recovering from addiction to cannabis is hard. So is trying to help someone caught in addiction. Both require psychological growth and demand behavioral changes on everyone's part: the person suffering from addiction, the family that suffers from watching a loved one grow more distant, teachers who lose a willing student, and peers who lose a friend. And yet, all this difficult change pays dividends that addiction is incapable of delivering, and in fact blocks.

While parents should not expect to find a system of prevention and treatment already integrated into schools, they should begin demanding it. Until that demand is heard, their children will continue to find unlimited access to cannabis but only limited access to treatment. The financial cost of an integrated prevention and treatment program for youth will be high for school counselors and outpatient and residential facilities, but the cost of delaying treatment and coping with the consequent lower quality of life will be higher. Taxpayers and parents should not be worried about the expense. A simple way of funding an entire youth prevention and treatment system is available. The cannabis industry is making big profits while avoiding the cost of mitigating the damage their products cause to youth and young adults. That does not seem fair, and a solution is discussed in the next chapter.

15 PUBLIC HEALTH
   AND POLITICS

Edward strode to the microphone on a mission. It was his opportunity to speak directly to California's Cannabis Advisory Committee and the head of the state's Bureau of Cannabis Control. He was given 90 seconds. A man of average height with a strong, athletic build, Edward's voice commanded attention without needing to be raised.

"I spent 5 years in prison for doing what I am legally doing today: selling cannabis to support my family. I have done everything you asked of me. I served my time. And now I have met all the requirements for starting a licensed dispensary. But the same police who arrested me to protect the public are failing to protect me when I am living as an honest citizen. Unlicensed and illegal cannabis dealers next door to my dispensary undersell me because they do not test for pesticides or collect the tax on cannabis that I have to. I have called the police and city council members. I have written to the Bureau of Cannabis Control and the state Attorney General's office, but it takes months before illegal stores are shut down. Then the dealers are released and open their store under a different name across the street. I call the police and city council members again, but it takes months again for anything to happen.

"I believe I went to prison because I am Black. But I believe dispensary owners of all races are not being served by law enforcement. If California wants legal cannabis businesses to be successful, you have to protect us from the illegal market. I think you can say

I have been fully rehabilitated as I stand here and plead with police to do their job, to serve and protect the public."

The room remained silent as Edward walked back to his seat with dignity after laying bare the difficulties of converting the underground world of illegal cannabis into a legitimate industry.

Few people thought about public health policies much until COVID-19 overtook the globe and sent us all into the shelter of our homes. Public health policy suddenly became a matter of life and death. Schools, jobs, shopping, and much of our entertainment were all put on hold, and the very lives of our parents, grandparents, and the most vulnerable among us were jeopardized. The US government's failure to respond with evidence-based information and clear guidance left many feeling like the grown-ups had forgotten to pay their light and water bills. Politicians did not take control and were not guided by common-sense science. Public health policy was confusing. As leaders downplayed the value of masks and social distancing, they wisely accelerated vaccine development but neglected to organize its distribution. Americans became divided about whether masks really work and who should be getting vaccinated first.

Although discussions about public health policy are generally considered boring and nerdy, there is no doubt that public health measures enacted by local, state, and federal governments have vastly improved the health and quality of life over the years. Without public health regulations, people would still be throwing their garbage and waste in the streets, burying their dead relatives wherever they please, working without proper safety precautions, and selling food, medicines, and other products with no guarantee of their purity or safety. Far fewer people would have access to medical care, and school children would not be required to have basic immunizations against measles, whooping cough, and polio. Smallpox would still exist at epidemic levels. Safe drinking water would be hard to find or would be a privilege afforded only by the wealthy. The world would be a more dangerous place and the average life span would be considerably shorter than we currently enjoy. Public health measures are among the most important actions that humans do cooperatively. Government is the mechanism by which good public health policies are developed and mutual cooperation is achieved.

We are living in a teachable moment. Its importance is acutely apparent, as is the damage that can be done by poor or inadequate public health policy decisions. Those of us in the field of addiction medicine have been aware of the damage ineffective drug policies have done for as long as we can remember. Prohibition of alcohol in the USA from 1920 to 1933 proved to be a disastrous public health effort. Not only was it generally ineffective but it also gave rise to organized and violent crime. Prohibition did reduce cirrhosis and alcohol-related death, but much of the public scoffed at the law and states began overturning its enforcement, as many are doing today with cannabis prohibition. The Noble Experiment, as alcohol prohibition was called, was bad policy and was eventually reversed in the USA, Finland, Russia, and elsewhere around the world, except in Muslim countries.

Cannabis prohibition has been equally unsuccessful. The plant grows everywhere, including in basements and attics under specialized grow lights. The law is scoffed at and violated by nearly half the US population. Current polls show that two-thirds of Americans favor cannabis legalization, and a constant stream of states are legalizing adult use, with more in the pipeline. Cannabis is still easily found in states where it is outlawed, as shown by the rate of past-month use among their adolescents being close to the national average.

Damage from Cannabis Prohibition

Cannabis prohibition was damaging to the nation in ways that differ from alcohol prohibition, which *only* made it illegal to manufacture, sell, or distribute alcohol. Wealthy individuals maintained a legal supply for their own consumption by buying the entire inventory of liquor stores before prohibition began. In contrast, cannabis was also illegal to buy, possess, and consume. As a result, not only was cannabis illegal, but any citizen caught with it was an outlaw. Jails and prisons eventually filled with cannabis felons, some of whom were busted for possessing only a couple of joints. Cannabis prohibition was enforced far more often and more severely on non-whites. The consequences of these felony convictions lasted longer than incarceration, including difficulty finding employment and loss of social welfare and education support. A criminal class, especially of Black males, was created because harsher penalties were imposed for Black and Latinx offenders than for whites for the same level of offense. We continue to pay the price today for these inequities, but ethnic minorities bear more of the burden than the dominant culture. For these reasons, states legalizing cannabis frequently include provisions to promote equity in the new cannabis industry. Public health policies and practices matter.

President Nixon politicized and weaponized cannabis prohibition when he created his War on Drugs. This contributed greatly to the escalating war against our own citizens for using drugs. While reducing the demand for any drug is a more effective public health strategy for mitigating harm than reducing the supply, reducing demand by locking up non-violent users does more harm than good. Treatment is more humane than incarceration and, ultimately, is more rehabilitating than prison. But politicians and voters usually see treatment as not being "hard" enough on drugs. Treatment is a "softer" approach. The War on Drugs called instead for a war on drug users. Over the years, police were equipped with military gear, and the DEA outsourced the War on Drugs into Central and South America by sending weapons and agents to lead attacks on drug producers in their countries. It would be an exaggeration to say this was all a waste, but perfectly fair to say it was unsuccessful enough to deserve serious rethinking.

Principles of Rational Cannabis Policy

A reasonable public health approach to preventing and treating harm from drug use would be to toss out our political ideologies and start again from the following basic principles and recognized realities:

1. The War on Drugs failed to protect us. Drugs originating both inside and outside the country continued to be widely available while the prisons filled, addiction remained a major health problem, and treatment remained fragmented and often unavailable to those most in need.

2. The legal and illegal cannabis industry is owned and run by adults. If adults did not desire access to cannabis, adolescents would have much greater difficulty obtaining weed.

3. Industries should be required to include the costs of repairing the damage done by their products in the price charged for them. This never occurred with the alcohol industry, leaving Big Alcohol to reap large profits while the costs of medical care caused by excessive drinking are largely borne by higher medical insurance premiums and the government's care of the poor.

4. Adult production and use of cannabis create an "attractive nuisance" for youth. The legal doctrine of

attractive nuisance holds a landowner liable for injuries to children if the injury is caused by a hazardous object or condition on their land that is likely to attract children who are unable to appreciate the risks posed. This principle is exemplified by the social responsibility we all have for removing doors from discarded refrigerators in order to protect young children from getting locked inside while playing with them. Under the attractive nuisance doctrine, the damage by cannabis to youth should be borne by the cannabis industry and its adult customers, and not the general, non-using public.

5. Youth currently have nearly unlimited access to cannabis but very limited access to treatment.

6. Regulating cannabis sales should eventually be able to suppress the illegal market, which is a major source of cannabis to youth.

7. Taxing cannabis sales could fund a system of prevention and treatment targeting the population at highest risk of harm from cannabis: adolescents.

8. States legalizing adult use of cannabis have generally found insignificant increases in the rate of adolescent use, although the rate of heavy use among those who already used may increase, which further emphasizes the need for cannabis tax revenue to fund effective youth treatment. However, the gold rush of new revenue is irresistible to states strapped for cash. Although Washington State has spent nearly half of its cannabis tax revenue on basic health services, too much of this revenue is siphoned off to general funds, road repairs, and early child development programs – all worthwhile projects, but they do not repair the damage done to youth by the cannabis industry.

Difficulties Establishing a Legal Cannabis Industry

Once it is agreed that neither of the extremes – total prohibition with intense policing and severe penalties, or unregulated, legal sales of cannabis – embodies the principles and fits the realities listed above, then a regulated market becomes the logical alternative. But deciding how to create a new industry in the face of an ongoing illegal market is very hard. Who will decide on the regulatory structure? Cannabis industry and business experts? Public health experts? Politicians? Lawyers? Police? Bureaucrats familiar with alcohol or tobacco regulations? The proper level of regulation will be a complex decision. Overregulation of some aspects of the new cannabis industry is as much a danger as underregulation of other aspects. Strong enforcement of regulations is expensive and raises fears of reactivating a new, thinly veiled War on Drugs with all of its racial biases. What should be done with people still in prison or weighed down by their past felony convictions, or even simple histories of arrest in a world where the Internet never forgets?

My membership on California's Cannabis Advisory Committee has given me a front-row seat to watch the growing pains of establishing a legal cannabis industry. Edward's difficulty getting law enforcement to shut down illegal dispensaries stealing his business is a perfect example of the problems facing legalization. Even before California legalized medical cannabis in 1996, law enforcement had begun turning a blind eye toward low-level cannabis offenses. Police were losing public support for arresting people for simple possession, and especially for preventing HIV/AIDS patients from treating their illness with cannabis. After legalization, California failed to regulate the medical cannabis industry in any meaningful way for the next 20 years. The law's vague indications for obtaining a "get out of jail free" medical marijuana card allowed virtually anyone to qualify for legally possessing cannabis. The police learned to look the other way and attend to more pressing duties.

A new reason to suppress the underground, illegal sale of cannabis emerged when recreational use of cannabis was legalized. License fees, the levying of excise and sales taxes on cannabis, and requirements for pesticide and strength testing all added to the cost of operation. Legal growers and retailers cannot compete with those operating outside the law. Enforcement has protected the alcohol industry very well. Moonshine liquor is rare, and illegal sales of beer or wine out of the trunk of someone's car are virtually non-existent. But cannabis is different. Early in its long prohibition, growers in California set up shop in the sparsely populated, rugged landscape of the Emerald Triangle: Humboldt, Mendocino, and Trinity counties. These "legacy" growers made a good living for two or three generations before their crops became legal. Now their profit margin has shrunk; the small farmer is being squeezed out of the legal market.

Only 10 percent of the cannabis raised in California today is sold legally in licensed dispensaries. The rest is either sold illegally in the state or shipped around the country. This underground segment of the cannabis industry is the biggest danger facing legal growers and sellers. The playing field is not level. Competition from illegal sales is fierce and impossible for licensed dispensaries to defeat. Only law enforcement can tilt the scales toward the legal market.

The job of law enforcement is further complicated by the tension between local control of dispensaries and delivery services. Following the Netherlands' model, the proposition legalizing adult recreational use (passed by 57 percent of California voters in 2016) enables counties and local jurisdictions to decide whether to permit cannabis dispensaries. However, as much of the cannabis is grown in Northern California and sold in the southern part of the state, the law permits cannabis to be transported through areas that do not permit retail sales in dispensaries. Citizens in counties without dispensaries still have the right to possess and use cannabis, so cannabis delivery services have expanded their range. A person living in a county that does not allow dispensaries can call or visit the website of a dispensary in a neighboring county, make a credit card purchase remotely, and have the cannabis delivered. As this does not differ in any significant way from asking a friend in the neighboring county to pick up an order on their way to visit you, such dispensary services have proliferated. However, what if a delivery person is robbed or delivers to someone under 21? Who has to bear the cost of prosecuting the crime? Trials are expensive. Counties in which cannabis is sold gain revenue by adding a tax to the sale, but the county in which the arrest occurred receives none of this revenue and has to pay police, prosecutors, and judges to prosecute delivery-related crimes. It should be no wonder that enforcement often remains lax. For example, since it was legalized in 2016, very few sting operations to investigate cannabis sales to underage customers have been conducted, despite this being a common tool used against alcohol sales to minors and cries by parent groups for increased enforcement.

Over- and underregulation is a common complaint of the industry and public health advocates, respectively. For example, California has a rigorous track and trace system that monitors the location of all cannabis plants, dried flowers, edibles, and concentrates. This Internet-based system follows cannabis from seed to sale, including during transport. Unfortunately, Internet connectivity in the remote Northern California hills is not always available, especially during the state's long wildfire season and intermittent power blackouts. The regulatory burden initially required growers to designate each seedling as either medical or recreational cannabis, even though they were often clones of each other. Nothing differentiates a plant as either medical or recreational, but each had to be designated as one or the other once a seed had sprouted, and never changed thereafter. This meant that retailers who ran out of a variety sold for recreational users could not shift inventory of the same variety sitting in their medical inventory, and vice versa. This illogical overregulation has now been changed. Furthermore, as growing cannabis and extracting oil for gummy edibles requires two separate licenses – cultivation and manufacturing – small operators must also be licensed to transport their crop from their field to a processing shed in a wheelbarrow. Then, they must file a track and trace report online to document the transport (by wheelbarrow), unless the Internet is down, in which case they need to fill out the proper paper form. Ultimately, there is a long distance between the theoretical value of many regulations and their practical implementation. All of this is a burden on the legal cannabis industry, costly in time, energy, and money that is not borne by the underground market.

At the same time, it is extraordinarily difficult to write public health regulations to protect youth that do not run afoul of freedom of speech and trade. Free enterprise naturally wants to be free of regulations and resists restrictions whenever it can. The stated goal of the cannabis industry is to "normalize" cannabis use. Public health advocates push back against the degree of normalization desired by the industry. Regulations requiring dispensaries to prominently post warnings of potential harm from cannabis are resisted on the flimsy basis of there not being sufficient scientific proof of health risks and arguments that the cannabis industry is being treated differently from other legitimate businesses. It is useful to recall the tobacco industry's uproar at being forced to include warning labels about the cancer-causing, addictive nature of their product to understand the force with which the cannabis industry fights against public health measures that decrease profits or interest in their product. As a result, a recommendation from the Public Health/Youth Subcommittee to the full Cannabis Advisory Committee to prohibit flavored THC vaping cartridges, with youth-attracting names like Bubble Gum and Butterscotch, has not been adopted by the committee as a whole. Members of the committee involved with the industry argue that "there is not enough science" to suggest that flavored vaping cartridges increase adolescent use or that flavored vaping is designed to attract youth, and they insist that "Adults like these flavors too." This opposition exists despite the fact that flavored tobacco vaping cartridges have already been banned in California for the same public health considerations.

Accepted public health regulations have also not been consistently implemented. For example, the original law legalizing cannabis also prohibited billboards on any road that crossed the California state line, which effectively meant they were banned along most major freeways. The Bureau of Cannabis Control decided to write regulations only to restrict billboards for the first 15 miles (24 km) within California's borders, but it was not clear who had responsibility for enforcing even this limited regulation. A lawsuit brought by an interested citizen was eventually necessary to strike down the Bureau's billboard restrictions. Cannabis dispensaries advertising on freeways can now lose their license. However, Weedmaps, which does not directly sell cannabis but runs a website for locating nearby dispensaries, does not have a license that can be revoked. Who is responsible for prosecuting their use of billboards, or does it somehow slip through a loophole as they are only advertising the website and not exactly advertising cannabis? Protecting the public's health against aggressive entrepreneurs is difficult, especially as public health agencies are not money-making endeavors. They rely on limited funding sources, unlike the industries they try to regulate.

I offer the above examples to illustrate the exquisite complexity involved in building a legal framework for the new cannabis industry. No regulatory agency can consider all the details, the endless implications and consequences of their regulations, and the basic practicality of all that could, or should, be regulated. My heart aches for all the struggling people like Edward, who are earnestly trying to follow the straight and narrow but are tripped up by government regulations still in their early trial-and-error stage, as well as for parents striving to protect their children from the attractive nuisance of legalized cannabis.

Principles for Creating a Regulated Cannabis Industry

My membership on California's Cannabis Advisory Committee has taught me five useful principles for legalizing cannabis. The first principle is to "go slowly." Even in the time it has taken me to write this book, two more states have legalized adult use of cannabis. Virginia is the most recent to reverse prohibition, but it will wait another 3 years before allowing sales to begin. This delay is prudent for three important reasons. First, it will provide sufficient time to create a new regulatory agency and carefully develop a regulatory framework after studying what has and has not worked in other states. Second, the delay before sales begin offers Virginia time to launch a public education program about the new law and guidelines for using cannabis safely. An educated public is the best assurance that their state will respond responsibly to the introduction of another legal, addictive drug. And third, "go slowly" means to start small and grow deliberately. This permits small growers to establish themselves in the new cannabis economy before permitting large corporations to enter. It also means permitting lower-THC cannabis flower and products before allowing higher concentrates. Ideally, it would be best to wait until adequate research has determined the safety and potential medical benefit of high concentrates. "Go slowly" also means monitoring the impact of different types of marketing as they are introduced. Delivery vans bearing bright signage driving through residential neighborhoods is not the best way for the new industry to begin.

The second principle is to create "one single regulatory agency." California's regulatory control was divided among the Bureau of Cannabis Control, the Department of Public Health, and the Department of Food and Agriculture. This made sense initially. For example, the Department of Food and Agriculture already knew how to regulate the use of pesticides and water usage. But this division meant that growers and dispensaries were required to correspond with multiple agencies for multiple different licenses. House regulation under a single agency simplifies matters and pulls experts from multiple disciplines into cooperating with each other. Five years after legalizing cannabis, California is now having to reorganize its cannabis regulation into a single, overarching department.

Third, "public health outweighs industry concerns." We must be careful to weigh regulations and advisory boards more heavily toward public health concerns than toward industry influence. It is much more difficult to rein the cannabis industry in than to loosen the reins as the industry matures. The California Cannabis Advisory Committee only had two health professionals among its 21 members when the Bureau first suggested we create subcommittees to focus on specific issues of importance.

They recommended eight subcommittees to discuss issues such as retail sales, licensing, distribution, banking, equity, and enforcement. I noted no mention of public health and youth issues, so I proposed a ninth subcommittee to recommend regulations to deal with these important concerns. I was flabbergasted when my motion was voted down, purportedly because a ninth subcommittee would overburden the Advisory Committee. When the majority of people in power are industry friendly, regulators will primarily cater to industry interests. They will argue that, without a thriving cannabis industry, there is nothing for public health advocates to regulate. When I mentioned that I would find it awkward and embarrassing if a reporter asked me to explain why the Advisory Committee had no Public Health/Youth Subcommittee, another committee member moved we reconsider the vote. As our meetings are open to the public and reporters were in attendance, the committee as a whole quickly voted to establish a subcommittee focused on regulations relevant to public health and youth. In the long run, the cannabis industry will only thrive if it acts responsibly by minimizing harm to youth; only public health professionals possess the expertise to guide regulations to achieve this goal.

Public input at Advisory Committee meetings was initially dominated by industry spokespeople and cannabis advocates. Those who are driven by financial gain and increased access are naturally going to attend and make their voices heard. Public health and youth concerns do not affect anyone's financial interests in the same way, and fewer organizations exist to attend Advisory Committee meetings. States legalizing cannabis need to actively elicit the public's input to balance the influence of the industry.

The fourth principle is "equity,", which means redressing the harm done by the War on Drugs, most often to minorities, and promoting opportunities for small business owners in an industry that is already prepared to coalesce into large corporate holdings. Edward is not alone in having his life derailed by laws and enforcement practices that society no longer supports. In addition, small legacy growers like those in Northern California are rapidly being squeezed out of the market. Towns in the Emerald Triangle are shuttering businesses as cannabis sales are flowing toward corporate owners.

Grower's licenses authorizing 10,000 ft^2 cultivation areas (a plot of only 100 × 100 ft, or 30 m^2) can support a small business and were made available in California 5 years before licenses for larger fields. However, corporations quickly bought multiple 10,000-square-foot licenses adjacent to each other to bypass that restriction. Economy of scale lowers the price and disadvantages small businesses. Edward and legacy farmers are small business owners, and equity means tilting regulations in their favor. Promoting equity disburses the industry among smaller owners. This disbursement should blunt the power of Big Corporate Marijuana, leaving politicians less dependent on their campaign contributions and freer to support public health goals.

The fifth and final principle is "youth first." When states begin contemplating legalization, the promise of a new tax revenue stream will dance like sugar plum fairies in politicians' heads. Everyone will begin fantasizing and then strategizing about where this pot of gold could be spent. Unless the principle of "youth first" is established at the outset, programs designed to help the youth harmed by cannabis will not be first in line to receive funding, and the opportunity to build an effective prevention and treatment system will be lost. Money will be siphoned off in dozens of directions, each arguably worthy and underfunded. As a result, the industry and the customers who support it will never be held responsible for repairing the damage done by its products. The cost of cannabis will remain lower and profits higher, all at the expense of youth unable to find adequate treatment. The states will continue having to foot the bill for their care and the needed social services. Unfortunately, spending tax revenue on drug-abusing youth remains a hard sell to the public and will require strong and dedicated leadership to be achieved.

Conclusion

COVID-19 has created a teachable moment about public health, and Edward raised important concerns about the process of legalizing cannabis. I may never see Edward again, but millions of Edwards live across our country. They teach us that the cannabis industry has been a part of every community for our entire lives and isn't going away. Legal or not, it is a fact of life. If we keep it illegal and try to suppress it with force, or if we simply ignore it, the cannabis industry will continue to outsource its damage (particularly damage to youth) to be paid by families and society at large. Instead, we can choose to regulate the industry, trust the vast majority of adults to use cannabis safely if given information about its risks, and use the tax revenue paid by those who use cannabis to support treatment for those who are harmed. If we position youth at the front of the line for education, prevention, support, and treatment when needed, I think we will be better off. This does not mean all problems will be solved, only that they will be lessened and more manageable. That would represent real progress. The legal cannabis industry needs to accept that it is no longer the unrestrained free enterprise it was during federal prohibition. It can only exist as a legal enterprise if it is a closely regulated industry.

EPILOGUE: THE FUTURE OF CANNABIS

Morris stood up at the end of our last therapy session. He was leaving the following day to return to his parents' home after being convicted of marijuana cultivation and sale. I had been treating Morris's anxiety as he felt the law's tightening grip around the sprawling cannabis business he had built. Proud of his success at managing such a large operation, he had arrogantly and deludedly believed that cannabis would be legalized before he was arrested. A defeated smile crossed his lips as he gravely shook my hand and said defiantly, "You know it's only a matter of time. I will be vindicated in the future." And he has been. We both understood the future of cannabis back then. What does the future look like now?

I turned 76 years old toward the end of writing this book. I am likely to see what becomes of cannabis in the next 5 years, and possibly the next 10. Much beyond that would be an extravagant gift, so I will end with a few speculations about the future of cannabis. Only time will tell whether I am prescient or dealing in mere fantasy. Either one would be amusing.

The story of cannabis has a great many twists and turns. Over the course of my lifetime, I have watched it leak out of the shadows occupied by jazz musicians and beatniks into the bright light with hippies dancing in San Francisco's Golden Gate Park, and then spreading throughout the youth culture at Woodstock and onto campuses, city street corners, and small towns across America. It became the younger generation's symbol against the Vietnam War and for release from the restrictive cultural norms of the 1950s. At the same time, for older generations, the influx of cannabis into society symbolized national decay and lawless chaos. Tens of millions of Baby Boomers scoffed at cannabis prohibition, despite over 20 million being arrested since it began in 1937, most merely for personal possession. Beginning in 1996 with the rebirth of medical cannabis in California, the country has softened its view of the plant and gradually taken on a more nuanced view that separates cannabis from harder drugs. The trend today is toward further liberalization, with momentum building toward national legalization of adult use. In late 2020, the US House of Representatives voted to decriminalize cannabis and to permit states to decide its legal status. While the Senate is unlikely to follow suit quickly, there are enough advocates among both its conservative and liberal factions to guarantee the issue will rise to the level of legitimate national debate. Over half of all adult Americans have tried cannabis and two-thirds support legalization, so the debate will be lively.

Largely because severe penalties were levied against cannabis users until recently, a schism developed in our national dialog about cannabis. Advocates of legalization feel they are fighting for their lives, or at least for their liberty. Opponents of legalization, however, have been influenced by politicians' tough rhetoric and feel they are fighting against the forces of cultural destruction and chaos. Now that decriminalization, medical cannabis, or full legalization have occurred in most states without apocalyptic consequences, perhaps the chasm between pro and con views can be narrowed or even replaced by a more pragmatic perspective. As an article of faith, I wrote this book with the belief that scientific objectivity can combine with understanding and respect for the lens of Cannabis Culture to create productive dialog. My goal has been to contribute less to debate in favor of more conversation – the mutual exchange of ideas and feelings.

Future of Cannabinoid Medication

Medically, several likely developments will revolutionize cannabis's role in treating disease. Scientists will continue to explore the large variety of molecules produced by the plant. Unlike the traditional framework of developing one drug for one specific disease, medicine will need to test multiple combinations of the different cannabinoids. What ratio of CBD to THC is optimal for different illnesses? Will the addition of other cannabinoids, or even terpenes, increase the safety and effectiveness of cannabinoid medications? Cannabis Culture extols the virtues of natural botanicals, believing that whole-plant preparations contain an ideal balance of components that has evolved over millennia. Whether the balance that best benefits a plant is the proper balance for treating human disease still needs to be researched. This painstaking work by cannabis medical advocates will continue, but it will likely continue to be underfunded. The large-scale clinical testing necessary for FDA approval is expensive, and pharmaceutical companies will be hard pressed to reap enough profit from developing medicines from the whole plant to fund clinical trials. The major source of funding for such studies will have to come from the federal government for research at the National Institutes of Health and as grants to university laboratories. As a result, an unproven anecdotal/folk medicine aspect to medical cannabis will continue for some time to come.

The more traditional approach to scientific investigation of botanical medicines is to isolate the essential ingredient and then play around with modifications, searching for stronger and safer alterations of the basic molecule. This is precisely the path that led from using foxglove tea to digoxin for heart failure, and from penicillin extracted from mold to a variety of other "cillins," such as ampicillin and amoxicillin. Pharmaceutical companies will be more willing to fund research and clinical trials of chemically altered versions of the original plant cannabinoids. There is big profit to be made by discovering new, more effective, and safer drugs to patent. For example, finding a THC analog that is a far more powerful pain reliever without producing THC's psychoactive high or addiction, if one can be created, would be a boon to humanity as well as to a drug company's bottom line. Researchers are already working on bringing about this future for cannabis.

As a dizzying array of FDA-approved cannabinoid medications become available, including those that selectively block aspects of our ECS's functions, the descendants of medical marijuana will migrate into traditional pharmacies. Physicians will routinely write prescriptions for cannabinoid-based medications to treat specific illnesses. They may even be seen drinking coffee from mugs displaying the logo of medications containing the latest alteration of cannabis's basic chemistry. In other words, cannabinoid medications will become more thoroughly medicalized and join the list of fully accepted pharmaceuticals. If, as current medical cannabis advocates claim, cannabis is real medicine, a shift into traditional medical practice will inevitably occur. Medical doctors will see manipulation of the ECS as a legitimate and obvious approach to treating many diseases, and they will expect to use preparations with known quantities of pure medication.

Medical cannabis dispensaries will be at a disadvantage after safer and more powerful versions of cannabinoids become available through a doctor's prescription. A move to permit the sale of herbal cannabis preparations in health food and vitamin stores will begin. This will further diminish the importance of medical cannabis dispensaries, and much of the accumulated experience regarding folk medicine's use of cannabis will shift into these more traditional venues, leaving dispensaries to cater more to social/recreational users, similar to today's liquor stores.

The original concept of medical marijuana will gradually fall into being seen as an anachronism, much as foxglove tea is today. This shift toward being an anachronism will be slow and never complete, as a community of people devoted to folk medicine remedies will continue to use whole-plant preparations, a throwback to earlier times. In scientific and medical circles, however, the medical use of cannabis will take an important, maybe even honored, place in the historical archives of botanical discoveries alongside foxglove, willow bark, and St. John's Wort.

Social/Recreational Use

Non-medical use of cannabis will continue unabated around the world for the indefinite future. The pleasure of being high is too great for its popularity to disappear. There will be efforts to regulate high-THC products, such as dabs and vaping cartridges, to reduce their potency, or at least to require inclusion of CBD to mitigate the negative side effects, but these efforts will encounter strong opposing winds. The libertarian belief that people should be free to put whatever they choose into their own bodies, combined with well-financed industry lobbyists, blind trust in the free market's ability to regulate itself, and the permanent existence of an illegal market for whatever the regulated market is prevented from providing, will make it difficult for public health advocates to put a cap on potency. To the most dedicated recreational users, if a little is good, more is better. Competition between cannabis growers and manufacturers will always spur the race to the top in order to sell more bang for the consumer's buck. Once adult use of cannabis becomes fully legal throughout the USA and many other countries around the world, Big Marijuana will become a very muscular and fierce competitor of Big Alcohol.

Efforts to merge the cannabis and alcohol industries will be both pursued and opposed. It is impossible to predict how this struggle will be resolved. Big Alcohol, Big Tobacco, and Big Pharma have already begun investing in Big Marijuana. Alcohol giant Constellation Brands, maker of Corona beer, invested $4 billion for a 38 percent stake in Canopy Growth, Canada's largest cannabis company. Anheuser-Busch, maker of Budweiser, has invested $100 million in a venture with Tilray, a Canadian medical cannabis company, to develop a non-alcoholic, THC-infused drink, perhaps giving new meaning to the slogan, "This Bud's for You." The corporate owner of Philip Morris and Marlboro has invested $1.8 billion in Canadian cannabis producer Cronos for a 45 percent share of the company. Irish pharmaceutical company Jazz paid over $7 billion for the leading cannabis pharmaceutical company GW Pharmaceuticals. A tsunami of money is rushing toward cannabis on a global scale. It is too soon to say if puny national governments will have enough power to regulate giant, transnational corporations to protect the kids in your town's local schools.

Governments will increasingly place treatment at the center of drug policy instead of relying on enforcement, first for cannabis and then for harder drugs, although reactionary forces will always push in the opposite direction. Portugal and the city of Vancouver are already leading the way by decriminalizing possession of all drugs for personal use while still prosecuting traffickers and dealers. As I ponder this continuing trend toward liberalization, my mind turns to Morris. While he did brazenly flout the law in his naiveté, he was not built for prison and would have been an easy victim if surrounded by hardened criminals. I lost track of Morris after he returned to Missouri. If convicted of a federal crime, he could still be in prison. If he has been released by now, how would the weight of his felony conviction still be disrupting his life? Although the law intends to be applied fairly, it rarely is. I cannot stop thinking that if he had been convicted under California law, he would now be out of prison, his record expunged, and perhaps he might even be back in the business he loved.

The vast majority of adults who use cannabis will do so responsibly, adolescents will continue to regularly get their hands on pot, and a minority of users will continue to become addicted. Drug treatment will remain an ever-green industry, although patients with CUD will never require as much attention as those devoted to alcohol, which is a much more damaging drug to body, brain, and society. Countries with a single-payer national health service will create coordinated systems for early intervention and treatment of adolescent cannabis use before the USA because of the fragmentation of healthcare produced by America's amalgamation of capitalism and medicine.

A controversy will develop around providing cannabis access to prisoners. Already suggested as a means of reducing prison violence, the prospect of allowing inmates to tolerate their captivity by getting high smacks of an official effort to discard human lives rather than rehabilitate them. However, the idea might reduce the harm done by more dangerous drugs easily smuggled into most prisons and the overly generous use of psychoactive medication for behavioral control. In cases where a pharmacological straitjacket must be used, cannabis is not the worst choice.

Drug-Free Enhancement of Endocannabinoid System Activity

The future of cannabis that intrigues me most is wrapped around a question for which there are currently only speculative answers: Why is the ECS hardwired into the brain's reward system? We know that all elements of our ECS, including anandamide and 2-AG, CB1 and CB2 receptors, and the DNA instructions for all the enzymes to synthesize and metabolize them, existed before primitive neural networks developed brains. It is only as brains evolved to integrate all of an organism's sensory inputs and to coordinate its body's actions that the nucleus accumbens appeared. This reward system guides animals toward increasingly clever means of survival. How did a connection between endocannabinoid and reward systems make animals more fit for surviving hostile environments? Why does rewarding ECS activity give an evolutionary advantage? Evolution has effective ways of eliminating dysfunctional genetic mutations, so this connection likely serves some useful purpose. The THC in cannabis would not be rewarding, and ultimately addicting, if the ECS it activates were not wired into the nucleus accumbens to produce reward. Why?

Multiple aspects of reward need to be understood. In the most objective psychological sense, reward simply means that an animal is more likely to repeat behaviors that activate the reward system. That which is rewarded tends to be repeated. This occurs without any reference to pleasure. The soft drink industry has learned that adding small amounts of caffeine does not necessarily lead more people to say they like the taste of their product, but it does increase the number who want it and thus continue buying it. Caffeine rewards the brain, and this leads to repetition. We drink more of a soda when it is slightly caffeinated. This illustrates a second function of our activated reward system. Not only do we repeat behaviors that activate reward, but we also feel motivated to repeat them. The reward system can be seen as bending motivation toward whatever activates it. Again, this does not necessarily involve pleasure in the way we normally think of it. For example, I have heard many alcoholics tell of going out late on a cold, rainy night to buy another bottle of liquor – a clear sign of urgent motivation – despite saying earnestly that they do not even like drinking any more.

Finally, in addition to repetition and motivation, the reward system does also contribute to the sensation of pleasure. As many people like to say, pleasure comes with a hit of dopamine (in the nucleus accumbens). While this is an oversimplification, it expresses the pleasure most cannabis users feel when THC's activation of the ECS increases dopamine in our reward center.

Why and how does any of this increase survival? The answer probably lies in looking at three basic activities known to activate the ECS: food, exercise, and sexual activity. Clearly, any animal that is able to eat regularly, exercises enough to remain fit, and has enough sex drive to reproduce has a good chance of survival. Our ECS evolved to sustain these basic healthy functions. In addition, the emergence of mammals, whose newborns possess a vital need to suckle soon after birth, depended on a high level of endocannabinoid activity to initiate feeding. As research shows, blocking endocannabinoid activity with rimonabant dooms newborn mammals to an early death.

Fascinating new directions will open as the public gains a deeper understanding of the brain's natural cannabinoid system. People who use cannabis already know the pleasant experiences it brings because THC increases activity in the ECS, including relaxation, novelty, vivid sensations, connectedness, forgetting negative experiences, and sometimes awe, joy, flow, laughter, and the creativity of connecting dots that typically lie outside the box of day-to-day thinking. Being high gives people a different experience of themselves and the world, which can create awareness of having lived too rigidly within a single default perspective. Learning this valuable lesson opens a person's mind to explore the world differently. The danger of relying on cannabis to achieve this is that some people end up endlessly and uncritically repeating the experience of getting high. The addictive potential of cannabis, some people's genetic susceptibility to addiction, and our lazy inclination to avoid the work of deeper psychological growth all combine to trap some people in a cycle of use that stalls further development.

In addition to the potential for addiction, scientific research has documented cannabis's negative impacts on cognition and emotions. As I have shown throughout this book, the impacts of too-frequent cannabis use result from four changes in the brain: chronic downregulation of cannabinoid receptors, reduced synaptic connections, loss of axon integrity, and hijacking of the brain's reward center. These cannabis-induced reductions in ECS functions, along with the negative effects of blocking the ECS with rimonabant, confirm that a healthy, active, well-balanced ECS is essential for physical, mental, and emotional health. Herein lies the likely reason that evolution hardwired our endocannabinoid and reward systems together. Health and wellness are supported by behaviors that sustain a baseline level of activity in our endocannabinoid chemistry. By pairing reward with endocannabinoid activity, we are motivated to repeat behaviors such as exercise and eating that keep us fit and fueled. Rewarding sexual activity ensures reproduction of the next generation, and rewarding newborns for suckling and both parents and infants for bonding physically and emotionally keeps the species healthy. While the ECS is not solely responsible for maintaining all these health- and survival-oriented behaviors, its proper balance is absolutely crucial to success. The phrase "necessary but not sufficient" perfectly describes the role of a well-balanced ECS for good mental and physical health.

Unfortunately, the unintended consequences of this hardwiring between the endocannabinoid and reward systems also created the potential for addiction when the cannabis plant was discovered. For the first time in history, stimulation of endocannabinoid activity from external sources became possible.

I believe we are on the cusp of learning to produce and value behaviorally induced endocannabinoid-based experiences as a primary source of pleasure and wellness. Just as people commonly speak of enjoying the endorphin high created by physical exercise and the "dopamine hit" that video games deliver, people will begin seeking the pleasure of an endocannabinoid high. Scientists have already shown that endocannabinoids circulating in the blood increase even more than endorphins in response to exercise. The runner's high may turn out to be mostly a cannabinoid-based experience. With increased science literacy, people will begin extolling the virtues of endocannabinoids as glibly as they now discuss the value of endorphins.

In the future, people will search for non-drug means to stimulate endocannabinoid-based experiences for physical and emotional relaxation. Behaviors designed to alter consciousness, vivify sensations, refresh perceptions, and produce a sense of awe through increasing endocannabinoid activity will be discovered and enhanced. Meditation, prayer, chanting, music, and the touch of massage are already known to increase endocannabinoids circulating in the blood. Special exercises and perhaps even biofeedback will be developed to further increase endocannabinoids. As-yet-unimagined technologies will be explored to balance or stimulate our ECS. Entrepreneurs will take advantage of the public's interest in endocannabinoid health, and fads will come and go.

Endocannabinoid System Deficiency

Cannabis Culture will be strengthened by rising interest in endocannabinoid health, and it will mistakenly advocate for the use of cannabis to support alleged deficits in endocannabinoids. Without solid scientific evidence, people will be encouraged to see their stress, anxiety, restlessness, boredom, and insomnia as symptoms of endocannabinoid deficiency, just as people with depression are told they suffer from a deficit of serotonin. The simplistic remedy for purported endocannabinoid deficiency will be to stimulate a flagging ECS with the right brand and amount of medical cannabis. The unfortunate result of this common-sense remedy will be to promote downregulation of receptors for which continued use of cannabis will be seen as the perfect antidote.

There is currently no proof that endocannabinoid deficiency is a real, naturally occurring syndrome. However, there is no logical reason why such a condition could not exist. In fact, genetic differences in the density of cannabinoid receptors have already been shown to exist, with significant impact on an individual's temperament. Psychiatry treats depression with medications designed to increase serotonin levels without a means of measuring whether the patient has an actual serotonin deficiency. Why should people suffering from stress, anxiety, restlessness, boredom, and insomnia not be treated similarly?

The answer is that cannabis has the ability to relieve these symptoms only transiently, at the cost of increasing their severity in the long run. Depression is not treated with medications that act as "super serotonin receptor activators" in the same way that THC is a "super cannabinoid receptor activator." The SSRIs used to treat depression work by prolonging the action of the brain's natural serotonin without leaving people feeling drug affected. Although some downregulation of serotonin receptors occurs with SSRIs, the increased level of serotonin more than compensates. THC, in contrast, more powerfully reduces cannabinoid receptors, compensates for down-regulation over a shorter period of time, and causes people to feel quite profoundly drug affected. If treatment is developed for symptoms believed to result from an inherent endocannabinoid deficiency, it will very likely be one that increases the level of the brain's naturally occurring anandamide and/or 2-AG, rather than directly stimulating receptors. This can be accomplished with medications that slow the metabolic breakdown of natural endocannabinoids. With increased understanding of the science of cannabis and the brain, the public will come to see that, while anandamide and 2-AG are natural parts of the brain and THC is a natural part of the cannabis plant, THC is not natural to the human brain.

Final Conclusions

Much lies ahead for the future of cannabis. The public will understand why maintaining a well-balanced ECS is important for good physical and psychological health. Behaviors supporting endocannabinoid strength and balance will become a part of wellness practices. Guided by this understanding, people will feel safe using cannabis as long as they stay within their brain's capacity to remain chemically balanced. If you "Know Your Limits," you will be safe.

As cannabis policy continues to relax in the USA and globally, legalization of adult use will lead the way toward a more rational drug policy in general. Prohibition always creates niche for criminal entrepreneurs and forces drug users underground in league with dealers. As a result, prohibition inevitably spawns a battle between law enforcement and the illegal drug industry, with huge monetary and political stakes. A few dealers and many users suffer, but enforcement never diminishes human desire. Instead, enforcement becomes its own industry within government bureaucracy. In the words of a respected colleague, the treatment and enforcement industries compete for the same raw material, so users are sorted out between prison and rehab, often based on their ethnicity and financial resources. This stalemate between enforcement and illegal drug dealers on the one hand and enforcement and treatment on the other can be ended with legalization and proper regulation. When drug users are only directed toward treatment, if necessary, enforcement can concentrate more effectively on illegal, organized operators. As a result, a nation's entire drug policy becomes more humane and potentially more effective at delivering treatment to those who need it. Treatment and recovery are the only ways in which demand for drugs can be reduced.

Cannabis legalization is the tip of the spear directed toward the failed but still popular War on Drugs. When cannabis legalization is successfully regulated, criminal violence around this soft drug will be virtually eliminated and treatment upon request will be adequately funded. This is not a utopian fantasy. There are still kinks to work out, but many states are already approximating success. The most serious barriers to success lie in the battle that already exists between Big Marijuana and the forces of public health. This battle will become much more intense over the next few years. Although many members of the cannabis industry, especially small legacy growers and serious patient advocates, understand that the health of their industry depends on not undermining the public's health, the large corporate interests that are starting to dominate will likely operate with the same money-induced lack of ethical code pervading Big Tobacco and Big Alcohol. Greed and self-interest, rationalized as the principles of free enterprise, will push the marketing of cannabis to its limits. Well-paid executives with teams of expensive lawyers will fight against anything that restricts profits, while underpaid public health gadflies and academics will mount scientific evidence and propose sophisticated policies to protect the public, but their progress in this David and Goliath struggle will be measured and slow. The same battles waged against Big Tobacco will be repeated with Big Marijuana. Déjà vu all over again. Gradually enlightened government action will be on the side of public health, just as it was in requiring warning labels on tobacco products and restricting cigarette smoking in public places. It will take decades for the government to find the proper balance between industry and public health interests. For the immediate future, the fortunes of the cannabis industry will be in the ascendency. Adequate government restrictions will probably have to wait until the industry has been well enough established to push illegal cannabis out of business to the same degree that moonshine no longer threatens the alcohol industry.

Legalization will spur society to take another small step toward maturity. With every adult having easy access to cannabis, public health messages will have to go beyond promoting fear of arrest and presenting warnings about unsubstantiated harms. Realistic reasons for caution will become the norm, but they will need to be described and explained honestly. More people will rely on science for factual information, and the evidence-based five signs of overuse will be used to teach people how to use cannabis safely. Scare tactics will be replaced by education that increases science literacy about cannabis and the brain.

I recognize that much of this is aspirational, but the effort to help people "Know Your Limits" is realistic. Anyone who has read to the end of this book has already taken a major step toward understanding how cannabis can be used safely, who should consider avoiding its use, and when their limits have been exceeded. It is up to each of us to be honest with ourselves. I can teach you what science has discovered about cannabis and the brain, and I can share my fascination about the mystique of cannabis. Only you can be honest with yourself. Godspeed.

ACKNOWLEDGMENTS

Jessica Papworth at Cambridge University Press encouraged this project from the beginning and shepherded it through to the end. This is the second time she has nursed one of my books through the publication maze and I deeply appreciate her consistently positive approach and ease of collaboration. Production editor Ruth Boyes and the entire CUP team provided expert and genuinely pleasant assistance. Three editors have ironed out my writing and deserve the reader's appreciation. My wife, Mary, bore the burden of reading the roughest drafts and letting me know where my prose was opaque and incomprehensible. Meredith Maran provided invaluable developmental suggestions, and Katie Lowery (clear.voice.tx@gmail.com) provided incredibly rapid turnaround with final text editing. The working relationship with all three is to be envied. Finally, the graphic designer Mary Osborn did heroic work with illustrations, given the author's extreme visual impairment.

Many colleagues have encouraged my development and writing. Special thanks to Dr. Mark Stanford for feedback on early drafts and help confirming several data points. Drs. Peter Banys and David Kan at the California Society of Addiction Medicine (CSAM) have provided challenging perspective over the years, and I am especially grateful for the opportunities provided by CSAM to appear at their conferences and for the opportunity provided by California's then Lt. Governor Gavin Newsom to lead the Youth Work Group of his Blue Ribbon Commission on Marijuana Policy Reform. I benefited from support by Dr. Bill Haning and Dr. David Smith, the latter of whom graciously agreed to provide this book's preface.

   Underlying everything I have learned about cannabis are patients who shared their experience and private worlds with me over the decades. I consistently admired how their courage pierced through their fear often enough to make fundamental changes in their lives. I remain honored and humbled by their trust.

GLOSSARY

2-AG (2-arachidonoylglycerol): a naturally occurring neurotransmitter that activates cannabinoid neuroreceptors.

Al-Anon: a mutual support group for those whose lives have been affected by a family member or friend's drinking or other drug use.

Amygdala: the brain area generating emotion, fight and flight, and novelty.

Anandamide: a naturally occurring neurotransmitter that activates cannabinoid neuroreceptors.

Antioxidant: a substance that prevents oxidative stress by scavenging free radicals.

Arachidonic acid: the fat molecule in cell membranes from which anandamide and 2-AG are synthesized.

Attractive nuisance: a dangerous condition that may attract children and risk their safety.

Axon: the long extension from a neuron cell body reaching out to downstream neurons.

Basal ganglia: a collection of neuron cell bodies lying beneath the surface of the brain and involved in the motor system (voluntary movement).

Bhang: a traditional intoxicating drink of India typically containing ground cannabis leaves and flowers mixed with milk or yogurt, water, and spices.

Big Marijuana: the outsized political and financial power of the cannabis industry.

Brain stem: an area at the base of the brain controlling involuntary functions such as breathing.

Bud: a cannabis flower, often dried and cured in preparation for smoking.

Budder: very high THC extraction from cannabis using volatile solvents.

Budista: a salesperson at a cannabis dispensary.

Budtender: a salesperson at a cannabis dispensary.

Butane hash oil (BHO): concentrated THC extracted from cannabis flowers and leaves by butane.

Cannabinoid: referring to cannabis-like qualities.

Cannabis Culture: the community of cannabis advocates based on beliefs about the meaning and value of experiencing cannabis, including spiritual, political, and economic dimensions.

Cannabis use disorder (CUD): formal diagnostic category for what the general public calls cannabis abuse, dependence and addiction, with specific criteria listed in the *Diagnostic and Statistical Manual of Mental Disorders*, used for medical, insurance, and research purposes.

CB1: a cannabinoid receptor found largely in the brain.

CB2: a cannabinoid receptor found largely throughout the body outside the brain.

CBD: the abbreviation for cannabinol, a largely non-psychoactive chemical in cannabis that modifies the impact of THC.

CBG: the abbreviation for cannabigerol, a non-psychoactive chemical in cannabis that is the immediate precursor of both THC and CBD.

Cerebellum: a highly organized collection of neuron cell bodies at the back of the brain involved with fine motor control and the sense of time.

Charlotte's Web: a cannabis plant variety with very high CBD and low THC used to treat severe childhood epilepsy.

Cingulate gyrus: an area of the cerebral cortex that helps regulate behavior, including error awareness and a sense of certainty.

Classical conditioning: a process of learning by associating a neutral stimulus (e.g. a bell) with a naturally occurring stimulus (e.g. food).

Compassionate Use Act: the 1996 proposition relegalizing medical cannabis in California.

Contracting: a process of formally outlining responsibilities and rewards between parent and child.

Corpus callosum: the large tract of axons interconnecting the left and right sides of the brain.

Cortex: an elaborately folder layer of neuron cell bodies covering the surface of the brain.

Cortisol: the body's primary stress hormone, secreted by the adrenal glands in response to signals from the hypothalamus and pituitary.

Couch lock: slang for the physical immobility that heavy cannabis intoxication can create.

CUD: the abbreviation for cannabis use disorder.

Dab/dabbing: a technique for inhaling vapor from concentrated cannabis resin by use of a device that rapidly heats the resin.

Decriminalization: removal of criminal penalties for cannabis use, although civil penalties such as fines similar to traffic infractions may still be levied.

Dendrite: a short extension from a nerve cell body with neuro-receptors that axons deliver neurotransmitter to at synapses.

Δ^9-tetrahydrocannabinol: the scientific name, referred to as THC, for the main psychoactive ingredient in cannabis.

Dispensary: a store that is the point of retail sale for cannabis products.

Double-blind studies: the gold standard for scientific research involving both administrators and consumers of a medication being unaware of its identity.

Downregulation: the reduction of neuroreceptors due to excess activation.

ECS: abbreviation for the brain's endocannabinoid system.

Edibles: cannabis products manufactured to be consumed orally and packaged as cookies, brownies, and candy, to name but a few examples.

Endocannabinoid system: the brain's system of natural THC-like neurotransmitters (e.g. anandamide and 2-AG), the enzymes to synthesize and break them down, and the unique cannabinoid neuroreceptors (CB1 and CB2).

Endogenous: of internal origin.

Entheogen: a psychoactive plant used in religious, spiritual, or ritualistic contexts.

Epidemiology: the branch of medicine that deals with the incidence and distribution of disease.

Epidiolex: an FDA-approved cannabis extract medication with a high CBD:THC ratio used to treat severe childhood epilepsy.

Executive functions: higher-order intellectual functions permitting abstraction, effective planning, mental flexibility, focused concentration and judgment.

Extinction: the fading of a classically conditioned response after no longer being rewarded.

Fight or flight: the sympathetic nervous system response triggered by perceived threat that prepares the body to fight or flee.

Frontal lobes: the site of executive functions; the last portion of the brain to mature.

Ganja: slang for marijuana.

Go/No-Go test: a test of impulsivity, measured by the ability to withhold responses.

Gray matter: the collection of nerve cell bodies.

Hashish/hash: concentrated oil from marijuana flowers.

Hemp: the cannabis plant, especially when grown for fiber.

Hippocampus: the brain area involved in learning and memory.

Homeostasis: the tendency of biological organisms to maintain stability in response to stresses.

Hypothalamus: the brain area regulating appetite and stress hormones.

Illicit: illegal.

Indica (*Cannabis indica*): one of the two main species of cannabis, which is short and stocky and is associated with a more sedating "body" high.

Joint: a marijuana cigarette, usually hand rolled.

Marijuana: the dried flower and leaves from female cannabis plants.

Mary Jane: slang for marijuana.

Masked faces protocol: a test of the brain's sensitivity to subtle emotional cues.

Munchies: increased appetite for comfort foods stimulated by THC.

Myelin: the fatty insulation surrounding axons.

Negative feedback: when the end product of a process reduces the stimulus that initiated that same process.

Nerve tract: a bundle of axons interconnecting areas of the brain.

Neuron: a nerve cell, consisting of the nerve cell body containing chromosomes made of DNA in the cell nucleus, dendrites receiving neurotransmitters, an axon, and synapses between an axon terminal and downstream neurons.

Neuroreceptor: proteins sitting in cell membranes that respond to chemical transmitters by stimulating or inhibiting a neuron's activity.

Neurotransmitter: chemicals that enter neuroreceptors to stimulate or inhibit a neuron's activity.

Novelty: the quality of being new or different.

Nucleus accumbens: a group of nerve cell bodies that reward behaviors that lead to increased dopamine.

Patent medicine: a non-prescription medicinal whose contents are incompletely disclosed.

Pot: slang for marijuana.

Reward center: the nucleus accumbens, the group of nerve cell bodies that increases behaviors that lead to an increase in dopamine.

Rimonabant: a chemical that blocks cannabinoid receptors.

Sativa (*Cannabis sativa*): one of the two main species of cannabis, which is taller than the indica species and is associated with a more energizing high.

Schedule I: the DEA's highest level of restriction on drugs deemed to have a high potential for abuse and no accepted medicinal value.

Sinsemilla: marijuana from unfertilized female cannabis flowers.

Shatter: a very high THC extraction from cannabis using volatile solvents.

Skunk: varieties of cannabis with very high THC, with a strong fragrance like that of skunks.

Spliff: a hollowed-out cigar filled with marijuana.

Stroop test: a measure of the ability to ignore distractions.

Student Assistance Program (SAP): a confidential support service for school students similar to Employee Assistant Programs.

Synapse: the short gap between axon terminals and dendrites that neurotransmitters cross to activate downstream neuroreceptors.

Temporal lobe: a lobe of the cerebral cortex sitting near the ear and critical for consciousness.

Terpenes: aromatic compounds found in many plants that are highly concentrated in cannabis and give the plant its characteristic, often pungent, fragrance.

THC: most psychoactive chemical in cannabis, primarily responsible for causing people to get high; abbreviation of Δ^9-tetrahydrocanabinol.

Upregulation: the return of neuroreceptors to their normal number after being downregulated.

Vaping: use of an electronic device for inhaling vaporized solutions containing nicotine or cannabis oil.

Wax: a very high THC extraction from cannabis using volatile solvents.

Weed: slang for marijuana.

White matter: a collection of axons running together.

FURTHER READING

BOOKS: GENERAL

Baum, D. (1997). *Smoke and Mirrors: The War on Drugs and the Politics of Failure*. New York, NY: Back Bay Books.

Cermak, T. L. (2003). *Marijuana: What's a Parent to Believe?* Ebook available on Amazon.

Elliott, S. (2011). *The Little Black Book of Marijuana: The Essential Guide to the World of Cannabis*, 3rd ed. New York, NY: Peter Pauper Press.

Gray, S. (ed.) (2016). *Cannabis and Spirituality: An Explorer's Guide to an Anciety Plant Ally*. Randolph, VT: Park Street Press.

Lee, M. A. (2013). *Smoke Signals: A Social History of Marijuana – Medical, Recreational and Scientific*. New York, NY: Scribner.

Pollen, M. (2001).*The Botany of Desire: A Plant's-Eye View of the World*. New York, NY: Random House.

BOOKS: SCIENTIFIC

Cermak, T. L. (2020). *From Bud to Brain: A Psychiatrist's View of Marijuana*. Cambridge, UK: Cambridge University Press.

Iverson, L. L. (2018). *The Science of Marijuana*, 3rd ed. New York, NY: Oxford University Press.

Solowij, N. (1998). *Cannabis and Cognitive Functioning*. Cambridge, UK: Cambridge University Press,

TOPICS

RAPHAEL MECHOULAM

1. Listen to an interview with the Godfather of Cannabis Research – Professor Raphael Mechoulam: www.youtube.com/watch?v=MW8GDs89AU4 (accessed July 16, 2021).
2. Read an interview with Raphael Mechoulam in: Conversation with Raphael Mechoulam. *Addiction*, **102**(6), 887–893 (2007).

https://onlinelibrary.wiley.com/doi/full/10.1111/j.1360-0443
.2007.01795.x (July 16, 2021).
3. Multiple videos of Raphael Mechoulam can be found on
    YouTube (www.youtube.com).

HISTORY

Brecher, E. M. (1972). Chapter 54. Marijuana in the New World.
In: *The Consumers Union Report on Licit and Illicit Drugs*. www
.druglibrary.org/schaffer/library/studies/cu/cu54.html (accessed
July 16, 2021).
Vipers & the Gage: Cannabis in the Jazz Age. Northern Standard online
article. www.northernstandard.com/vipers-the-gage-cannabis-in-
the-jazz-age/ (accessed July 16, 2021).

SET AND SETTING

Hartogsohn, I. (2016). Constructing drug effects: a history of set and
setting. *Drug Science, Policy and Law*, **30**. https://journals.sagepub.com
/doi/full/10.1177/2050324516683325 (accessed July 16, 2021).

COMPARING CANNABIS AND TOBACCO SMOKE

Henry, J. A. (2003). Comparing cannabis with tobacco: smoking cannabis, like smoking tobacco, can be a major public health hazard.
British Medical Journal, **326**(7396): 942–943. www.ncbi.nlm.nih.gov
/pmc/articles/PMC1125867/ (accessed July 16, 2021).

EFFECTS OF MARIJUANA ON THE LUNG

Tashkin, D. P. (2013). Effects of marijuana smoking on the lung.
Annals of the American Thoracic Society, **10**(3), 239–247. www
.atsjournals.org/doi/pdf/10.1513/AnnalsATS.201212-127FR
(accessed July 16, 2021).

MR. X, BY DR. SAGAN

1. https://coloradocannabistours.com/blog/news/carl-sagan-was-
    mr-x/ (accessed July 16, 2021).
2. Article written by Carl Sagan in 1969 for publication in
    Marihuana Reconsidered, 1971: http://marijuana-uses.com/mr-x/
    (accessed July 16, 2021).

ILLEGAL DRUG USE STATISTICS

SAMHSA National Survey of Drug Use and Health: www.samhsa.gov
/data/sites/default/files/reports/rpt29394/NSDUHDetailedTabs2019/
NSDUHDetTabsSect1pe2019.htm (accessed July 16, 2021).

NATIVE AMERICAN AND CANNABIS CULTURE'S PERSPECTIVE ON CANNABIS AS MEDICINE

Wolf, J. "Medicine" in the Native American way of thinking. Facebook
article. https://m.facebook.com/nt/screen/?params=%7B%22note_id%
22%3A888240545042396%7D&path=%2Fnotes%2Fnote%
2F&refsrc=deprecated&_rdr (accessed July 16, 2021).

CANNABIS AND SPIRITUALITY: A HISTORY

Saunders, N. (2021). The spiritual history of marijuana . . . revealed! Way
of Leaf online article. https://wayofleaf.com/blog/the-spiritual-history
-of-cannabis (accessed July 16, 2021).

CURRENT STATE OF EVIDENCE FOR MEDICAL CANNABIS

National Academies of Sciences, Engineering, and Medicine (2017). *The
Health Effects of Cannabis and Cannabinoids: The Current State of Evidence
and Recommendations for Research*. Washington, DC: National
Academies Press. www.ncbi.nlm.nih.gov/books/NBK423845/
(accessed July 16, 2021).

CBD MARKET ANALYSIS

Dorbian, I. (2019). CBD market could reach $20 billion by 2024, says
new study. Forbes online article. www.forbes.com/sites/irisdor
bian/2019/05/20/cbd-market-could-reach-20-billion-by-2024-says-
new-study/#782cef4549d0 (accessed July 16, 2021).

TESTIMONIALS AND MARKETING

"Take it from me" – why testimonials are so effective. Strategic Factory
online article, 2017. https://strategicfactory.com/about-us/blog/take-
it-from-me–why-testimonials-are-so-effective.html (accessed July 16,
2021).

THE DISCOVERY OF CBD BY ROGER ADAMS

Wood, J. (2020). Roger Adams, the man who "discovered" CBD. Zebra CDB online article. https://zebracbd.com/blogs/cbd-education/roger-adams-discovered-cbd (accessed July 16, 2021).

CROSS-SECTIONAL STUDY OF CANNABIDIOL USERS

Corroon, J. and Phillips, J. A. (2018). A cross-sectional study of canna-bidiol users. *Cannabis Cannabinoid Research*, **3**(1), 152–161. www.ncbi.nlm.nih.gov/pmc/articles/PMC6043845/ (accessed July 16, 2021).

THE STRESS RESPONSE

Understanding the stress response. Harvard Health Publishing online article, 2020. www.health.harvard.edu/staying-healthy/understanding-the-stress-response (accessed July 16, 2021).

CBD AND DIABETIC RETINOPATHY

Liou, G. I., El-Remessy, A. B., Ibrahim, A. S., et al. (2009). Cannabidiol as a putative novel therapy for diabetic retinopathy: a postulated mechanism of action as an entry point for biomarker-guided clinical development. *Current Pharmacogenomics Personalized Medicine*, **7**(3), 215–222. www.ncbi.nlm.nih.gov/pmc/articles/PMC2955420/ (accessed July 16, 2021).

THE GATEWAY THEORY: AN ABSTRACT

Van Gundy, K. and Rebellon, C. J. (2010). A life-course perspective on the "gateway hypothesis". *Journal of Health and Social Behavior*, **51**(3), 244–259. www.meta.org/papers/a-life-course-perspective-on-the-gateway/20943588 (accessed July 16, 2021).

PUBMED

The US government offers free access to abstracts of the world's medical literature through its website https://pubmed.ncbi.nlm.nih.gov, or just Google "PubMed." With a little prac-tice, you can quickly search for detailed topics. For example, typing in the word "cannabis" and additional details such as "multiple sclerosis muscle spasms" in the query box immediately pulls up a list of relevant articles, with the first abstract describing a trial of cannabis extracts in the treatment of multiple sclerosis muscle spasms. PubMed is an invaluable resource for exploring the latest medical and scientific research.

FIGURE SOURCES

Figure 2.1   Photo by Eldad Carin (iStock by Getty Images).

Figure 2.2   This is in the public domain.

Figure 2.3   Photos of leaves by rgbspace (iStock by Getty Images). Plant illustrations based on image from: R. Quinones (2014). What is the difference between indica and sativa? theweedblog.com. https://bit.ly/3jMOzuj

Figure 3.1   Figure created by Mary Osborn, Graphic Designer, www.mosborndesigns.com.

Figure 3.2   Image based on Katona, I., Sperlágh, B., Sík, A., et al. (1999). Presynaptically located CB1 cannabinoid receptors regulate GABA release from axon terminals of specific hippocampal interneurons. *Journal of Neuroscience*, **19**(11), 4544–4558.

Figure 3.3   Image based on Katona, J., Sperlágh, B., Sík, A., et al. (1999). Presynaptically located CB1 cannabinoid receptors regulate GABA release from axon terminals of specific hippocampal interneurons. *Journal of Neuroscience*, **19**(11), 4544–4558.

Figure 3.4   National Institute for Drug Abuse (NIDA) (2021). How does marijuana produce its effects? https://bit.ly/3AxiygS

Figure 5.1   Johnston, L. D., Miech, R. A., O'Malley, P. M.,
              et al. (2018). *Monitoring the Future National
              Survey Results on Drug Use: 1975–2017: Overview,
              Key Findings on Adolescent Drug Use*. Ann Arbor,
              MI: Institute for Social Research, The
              University of Michigan.
Figure 5.2   Based on data from Johnston, L. D., O'Malley,
              P. M., Bachman, J. G. and Schulenberg,
              J. E. (2011). *Monitoring the Future National Survey
              Results on Drug Use, 1975–2010: Volume I,
              Secondary School Students*. Ann Arbor, MI:
              Institute for Social Research, The University
              of Michigan.
Figure 5.3   Miech, R. A., Johnston, L. D., O'Malley, P. M.,
              et al. (2020). *Monitoring the Future National
              Survey Results on Drug Use, 1975–2019: Volume I,
              Secondary School Students*. Ann Arbor, MI:
              Institute for Social Research, The University
              of Michigan.
Figure 5.4   Substance Abuse and Mental Health Services
              Administration (2017). *Key Substance Use and
              Mental Health Indicators in the United States:
              Results from the 2016 National Survey on Drug Use
              and Health (HHS Publication No. SMA 17-5044,
              NSDUH Series H-52)*. Rockville, MD: Center for
              Behavioral Health Statistics and Quality,
              Substance Abuse and Mental Health Services
              Administration. www.campusdrugprevention
              .gov/sites/default/files/files/2017%20NSDUH
              %20Findings.pdf
Figure 5.5   Substance Abuse and Mental Health Services
              Administration (2017). *Key Substance Use and
              Mental Health Indicators in the United States:
              Results from the 2016 National Survey on Drug Use
              and Health (HHS Publication No. SMA 17-5044,
              NSDUH Series H-52)*. Rockville, MD: Center for

Behavioral Health Statistics and Quality, Substance Abuse and Mental Health Services Administration. www.campusdrugprevention.gov/sites/default/files/files/2017%20NSDUH%20Findings.pdf

Figure 7.1   Pertwee, R. G. (1997). The therapeutic potential of cannabis and cannabinoids for multiple sclerosis and spinal injury. *Journal of the International Hemp Association*, **4**(1), 1, 4–8. ©American Neurological Association.

Figure 11.1   Budney, A. J., Vandrey, R. G., Hughes, J. R., Thostenson, J. D. and Bursac, Z. (2008). Comparison of cannabis and tobacco withdrawal: severity and contribution to relapse. *Journal of Substance Abuse Treatment*, **35**(4), 362–368.

Figure 12.1   Winters, K. C. and Lee, C.-Y. S. (2008). Likelihood of developing an alcohol and cannabis use disorder during youth: association with recent use and age. *Drug and Alcohol Dependence*, **92**(1–3), 239–247.

INDEX